christian YOGA

Super Advanced Course
Number One
Lessons 1 to 12

SWAMI YOGANANDA

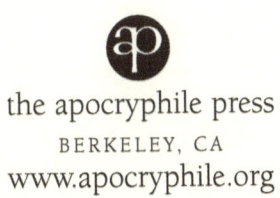

the apocryphile press
BERKELEY, CA
www.apocryphile.org

apocryphile press
BERKELEY, CA

Apocryphile Press
1700 Shattuck Ave #81
Berkeley, CA 94709
www.apocryphile.org

Originally published by the Yogoda Sat-Sanga Society.
Apocryphile Press Edition, 2007.

Printed in the United States of America
ISBN 1-933993-50-2

Super-Advanced Course No. 1

•••❖•••

Lesson No. 1

•••❖•••

CHRISTIAN YOGA AND THE HIDDEN TRUTHS IN ST. JOHN'S REVELATION INTERPRETED ACCORDING TO INTUITIONAL EXPERIENCE

By

SWAMI YOGANANDA

•••❖•••

This sacred lesson is meant only for the devoted Yogoda
student who would, untiringly and unceasingly,
seek God until he finds Him

•••❖•••

Published By
YOGODA SAT-SANGA SOCIETY
3880 San Rafael Avenue
Mount Washington
Los Angeles, Calif.

The spinal passage and the seven astral doors of escape, including the medullary door through which the soul can fly to the Spirit.

Of all the books in the Bible, *Genesis* and *Revelation* are the two most important. The first chapter of *Revelation,* which is the basis of this lesson, contains the hidden truths of Christian metaphysics and Hindu Yoga as revealed through the intuition of St. John.

Revelation means "that which has been revealed." How? Not through intelligence but through intuition. This lesson is merely a spiritual forecast; as you proceed to the highest pinnacle of understanding, these truths will be revealed to you by the light of your intuition.

What is the difference between understanding and intuition? Understanding depends upon the senses for knowledge; intuition brings direct perception of truth. When you see a rope in the dark, you may think you are seeing a snake. Your inferences are often mistaken, because your intelligence can reach its conclusions only through the data supplied by the senses. If the senses mislead you, your inferences are necessarily wrong. Intuition, on the other hand, does not depend on intelligence or sense perception. At times you have a feeling that something is going to happen. You do not hear or see anything on which to base the expectation, but it happens. This is popularly called a "hunch." Try to change your "hunch" to controlled intuition by meditation. Thus it will become a scientific factor.

In the past, Christianity has remained aloof from Hindu religion. Real Christianity is not to be blamed for this; it

1

is "churchianity" which is responsible for paralyzing rational religious thinking. Attending churches or temples of God-worship is a good thing, but in itself does not prove actual knowledge of God. Actually knowing God is another matter. Christianity will become the stronger for discarding dogmatic beliefs and supplementing its appeal through a study of the universally true, intuitionally received spiritual experiences of the Hindu savants.

Many religious teachers are but "spiritual victrolas." They grind out sermons without experiencing the truths contained in them. St. John did not deliver sermons he did not realize. He wrote what he saw, felt, and learned intuitively during his meditations. Without knowing and practicing some great method of meditation (as the fifth Yogoda lesson), it is impossible to experience the mysteries of life, or to know all the intricacies of the human body, the soul, and the cosmos.

So the hidden truth in *Revelation* is intuition-discovered and will be found to be universally acceptable. Whether you are a Christian, Jew, Buddhist, or Mohammedan—if you study the truths that are interpreted here for you, not only through the intellect but through intuitive meditation, you will find that they agree with the essence of your own religious teachings.

St. John's *Revelation* can be understood and known only by Christian metaphysicians and Yogis. Jesus Christ was an Oriental and a Yogi.[1] A document found in a Tibetan

[1] Yogi: One (man, woman, or child) who unites himself or herself scientifically with God through Yoga methods (art of God-contact).

2

monastery proves that during His unknown life, between His twelfth and thirtieth year, He was in India and conferred with the wise men of the East (India) about the mysteries of the inner life, returning the visit they paid Him at His birth.

A detailed account of Jesus' visit to India can be found in a book entitled *The Unknown Life of Christ,* by Nicholas Notovitch. This Russian having heard of the document regarding Jesus, or *Issa,*[1] in the possession of Tibetan monks or lamas, went to Tibet to verify the report. He definitely established the fact of Jesus' visit to India during the time of His disappearance from Asia Minor. Therefore, Jesus taught the oriental, practical Christianity based on inner realization.

Modern Christianity, in spite of its moral and socioreligious foundation, lacks the expressions which come from self-realization of truths. Occidental Christians generally want salvation by proxy. The average Christian deems it sufficient to go to church regularly and to read the Christian Bible occasionally, though mechanically, forgetting to practice in daily life what he has heard and read. Your belief alone does not make you a Christian[2]; it is your realization of the Christian truths that does. If you study these lessons faithfully, you will be reborn spiritually and may call yourself a Christian Yogodan, or a Christian realist, or a true Brahmin.[3]

[1] *Issa:* Sanskrit, meaning *Lord.*
[2] Christian: One who has Christ Consciousness.
[3] Brahmin: Originally, one who has been reborn spiritually. The supreme teacher recognized only two castes: the Sudras (those bound to the body) and the Brahmins (those having attained Brahma—or God Consciousness).

Intuitional study of the scriptures results in tolerance through realization of the fundamental unity underlying all faiths, whereas arrogant, purely intellectual study of the scriptures is productive of argumentation and dissension. In other words, the latter reveals but the *outer* shell of truth, whereas the former discloses truth's *inner and outer* aspects simultaneously. Study the scriptures after meditation, when the intuitive state is predominant.

The seven Spirits.   St. John did not read a library full of books in order to write the book on Revelation. Jesus conferred with the Hindu Yogis on the universal art of Yoga (the art of human salvation). St. John, the beloved disciple of Jesus, received revelation after experiencing contact with the seven reflected spirits of God (Christ Consciousness and the six reflected spirits before the throne of His omnipresence. See *Revelation* 1:4 below.) St. John felt Cosmic Consciousness not only in his physical, astral, and ideational bodies, but also in the physical, electrical, and ideational universes before he ventured to write about the revealed truths. Many people try to teach after reading a few occult books. One is qualified to teach only after he has actually experienced metaphysical truths and has felt his consciousness beyond the body.

The four-caste system, which is of comparatively recent origin, recognizes the following castes:

    (1) Sudras (laborers)   (3) Vaisyas (merchants)
    (2) Kshatriyas (warriors)   (4) Brahmins (priests)

Under this system, children automatically take the caste of their parents. Originally, caste was based on different qualities.

4

To know truth, you must experience it in your own consciousness. *The Hindu Yogis and Swamis*[1] *practicing Yoga, or the science of oriental Christian metaphysics, have given almost identical descriptions in Yoga books of all that has been recorded by St. John from his inner experiences. This proves the influence of Hindu Yoga on the teachings of Christ.* Besides, there is only one truth, and there can be no fundamental difference among those who have realized it, whether they be Hindus or Christians. The moon presents the same face to all, and the one truth must likewise appear the same to all who have really lived it.

Revelation is the true record of St. John's intuitional experiences. Remember, this *Revelation* is true and will be found true not only by Christians, but by all so-called believers and unbelievers who follow the universal path to God. I am speaking from personal experience, and if you practice what you are studying, you will feel what I felt. According to the inner revelation of St. John and the Hindu Yogis, I am giving you a glimpse of the inner meaning contained in some passages in the first chapter of St. John's *Revelation*. We find in the tenth to twentieth verses of this chapter the most important record of spiritual experience and description of inner astral anatomy.

A condensed interpretation of this chapter follows:

Revelation 1:1 *The Revelation of Jesus Christ, which God gave unto him, to shew unto his servants things which must shortly come to pass; and he sent and signified it by his angel unto his servant John:*

[1]Swami: One who has achieved self-mastery and is endeavoring to attain perfection through renunciation.

5

Revelation 1 :2   *Who bare record of the word of God,*
                      and of the testimony of Jesus Christ,
and of all things that he saw.

St. John wrote only of that which he experienced while
he was listening to the Cosmic Sound of Om or the Word of
God and of the Christ—or Jesus Consciousness present in
the Cosmic Sound.   (See *Revelation* 1:10 **below.**)

The *angel* mentioned in *Revelation* 1:1 is intuition—a
conscious force within St. John—which bore testimony of
the truth coming from the vibration of *Cosmic Consciousness*[1] *and Christ Consciousness*[2] *(Word of God).*

Revelation 1 :4   . . . *the seven Spirits which are before
                      his throne* . . . refers to the seven mani-
festations of God in creating man.

All creation is divided into three macrocosmic and three
microcosmic manifestations.   When God brought forth
creation, His manifestations took the form of three universal
spirits and three macrocosmic objects.   The macrocosmic is
the whole—the ocean, and the microcosmic represents the
unit—the wave.

Manifestations of   There are six *subjective* manifesta-
the Spirit.   tions of the Spirit, reflected in its six *ob-*
                      jective manifestations:

Three microcosmic objects: Idea; cosmic energy; physical
cosmos;

[1]Cosmic Consciousness: God, the Father, or the Consciousness beyond all
creation.

[2]Christ Consciousness: The Consciousness in all vibratory creation.

6

Three macrocosmic subjects: The ideational Cosmic Architect; the astral Cosmic Engineer; the Builder of the gross cosmos.

Three microcosmic objects: Idea body; astral body; physical body;

Three microcosmic subjects: The ideational-body Creator; the astral-body Creator, and the Creator of the physical human body.

In all of the six macrocosmic and microcosmic objects, the Spirit is present as six subjective forms of consciousness or as one reflected Christ Consciousness. There is only one reflected Spirit, *the only begotten son,* called Christ Consciousness, which is the seventh manifestation, reflected in all objective creation. In the six objects the Spirit is reflected as six subjective spirits, and these six, as one reflection in all objective creation, are Christ Consciousness. This is the meaning of *the seven Spirits which are before his throne.*

Revelation 1:5   *And from Jesus Christ, who is the faithful witness, and the first begotten of the dead, and the prince of the kings of the earth . . .*

Christ or Jesus Consciousness is experienced as the princely supreme force governing all other potent material forces, when one first enters the spiritual kingdom by leaving his vitally suspended physical body. This is what is meant by *the first begotten of the dead and the prince of the kings of the earth.* Christ Consciousness perpetually witnesses all changeable creation governing all matter—each atom. As you meditate and rest from the astral, physical, and ideational bodies, your first perception is Christ Consciousness. You must rise beyond your several bodies before you can attain Christ Consciousness. St. John, after he experienced the truth by contacting Christ Consciousness lying beyond these three bodies and the six spirits, revealed this truth in this chapter of *Revelation*. God Consciousness transferred the universal truth through intuition to man.

Revelation 1:10	
The Cosmic Sound, or	I was in the Spirit on the Lord's day
Cosmic Trumpet, or the voice of	and heard behind me a great voice, as of
many waters, or Om, or Amen, or the Word.	a trumpet,[1]

Revelation 1:11   Saying, I am Alpha and Omega, the first and the last: and, What thou seest, write in a book, and send it unto the seven churches . . .

That is very clearly expressed. *In the Spirit* means within St. John's consciousness. (See the fifth Yogoda lesson.) St. John was approaching the Spirit—leaving the realm of matter, *i.e.*, the body and the material senses. He described vividly the experiences which he had as he entered the Infinite. He perceived his soul behind the ego (described as *me*) and the material consciousness and subconsciousness,

[1]Compare *Yoga Aphorisms* of the Hindu sage Patanjali: *The symbol of Spirit is Aum (Om), the Cosmic Sound.*

8

and through the finer perception of the soul he heard the Cosmic Sound manifesting Itself as trumpet sound, emanating from all vibratory creation. The trumpet was *Saying, I am Alpha and Omega*. Can trumpets speak? Not literally, but the Spirit can signify a meaning through trumpets or vibratory sounds. Whenever you hear that Cosmic-Trumpet Sound, you are hearing the Aum creative —preservative—destructive vibration. This vision and conscious experience of Cosmic Sound urged him to transmit his knowledge to the world through spiritual centres and churches where people seek God and His mysteries.

Revelation 1:12 The seven seals, or the seven chakras, or the seven golden candlesticks, or spiritual dynamic centres in the spine as described in the Yoga books.

And I turned to see the voice that spake with me. And being turned, I saw seven golden candlesticks;

St. John said in the tenth verse that he *was in the Spirit*; hence, when he spoke of *being turned*, he did not refer to bodily motions. He fixed his attention upon, and became one with, the voice which *spake* or vibrated within him, and as he stayed in that vibratory sphere he perceived the seven golden astral doors of escape which lay within his physical body. The physical and astral bodies are the bodies of energy. How are they connected? The physical body is attached to the astral body by seven candlestick-like vibratory seals. Energy flows into the spine through the physical body. Just as electricity flows into the bulb through

9

a wire passage, so the Cosmic Force flows through the medulla into the spine and its seven centres; into the body and its five sense lamps. The astral body of the life force is knotted to the physical body by seven golden candlestick-like burning seals.

What is the meaning of *candlestick*? In this book two terms have been used, *stars* as well as *candlesticks*; the former are the lights and the latter, the receptacles. *Angel* means *star*, and *church* also means receptacle.

The seven centres of light for the outgoing current are:

The mystery of the seven stars or lotuses.

(1) Thousand-petaled lotus star (seat of the beautiful, condensed, lotus-like, thousand-rayed life current performing the thousand-and-one functions in the body): Bliss-ether in which God and the angels abide; main dynamo. Cosmic energy enters the body through the medulla but is stored in, and distributed by, the whole brain;

(2) Medullary centre [seat of the two-rayed lotus star of life force (positive-negative current)]: Super-ether in which thoughts and the life force move;

(3) Cervical centre (seat of the sixteen-rayed lotus star of life force): Ether through which sounds and electrons travel;

10

(4) Dorsal centre (seat of the twelve-rayed lotus star of life force): Air (vitality);

(5) Lumbar centre (seat of the ten-rayed lotus star of life force): Fire (inner life energy);

(6) Sacral centre (seat of the six-rayed lotus star of life force): Water (circulation);

(7) Coccygeal centre (seat of the four-rayed lotus star of life force): Earth (the gross flesh).

The spinal cord may be likened to a wire. In it are located these seven centres of light which are the subcentres for the conduction and distribution of life current throughout the body. The body is nothing but a condensation of this spinal energy. Just as invisible hydrogen and oxygen atoms can be condensed into visible vapor, water, and ice, so light can be transformed into body which is nothing but frozen energy. You must lose all fear of sickness and accidents; as your body is nothing but energy, it cannot be harmed. When you realize this, you will be free.

The seven centres are the *churches* or *candlesticks*, and the seven *stars* are their dynamic radiating currents. *The Cosmic Energy enters through the medulla to be stored in the brain, whence it descends into the seven centres, feeding*

11

the seven elements[1] of which the body is composed. When these seven lights are withdrawn from the body in death, the body disintegrates.

In passing from the consciousness of the body to that of the Spirit, one experiences these seven sub-dynamic doors of energy fixed in the astral cerebrospinal axis. *The soul must leave the physical, astral, and spiritual bodies through the seven astral doors in order to reach, and merge into, the Spirit. After it lifts its consciousness from the physical body, it must unlock, and pass through, the seven astral doors in the spine.*

The Yogoda student, in the third lesson, first contracts the Cosmic Vibration. This is the first state of meditation. In the next higher state of meditation (see fifth lesson), the Yogi lifts his attention from the body. It is then that he perceives the *seven golden candlesticks* or seven astral doors of escape in the spine and falls as dead as his energy is switched off from the body.

Revelation 1:13   *And in the midst of the seven candle-sticks one like unto the Son of man,*

Golden girdle or   *clothed with a garment down to the*

astral radiation.   *foot, and girt about the paps with a golden girdle.*

St. John speaks of the form of the astral body as something similar to the *Son of man,* or the physical body which is born of man, or matter. He describes the astral body as built around *the seven candlesticks* or seven centres of golden life force, describing it as *a garment down to the foot* (the

[1]Bliss-ether, super-ether, ether, air, fire, water, and earth.

12

entire astral nervous system woven with filaments of nerve currents like a garment). The *golden girdle, about the paps,* or the swelled astral radiation, is the golden halo which surrounds, girdles, or spreads out around, the entire astral body. By looking steadily with unblinking eyes at the entire outline of one's body, one can see a vapor-like astral radiation—an astral aureole.

Revelation 1:14   *His head and his hairs were white like wool, as white as snow; and his eyes were as a flame of fire;*

Revelation 1:15   *And his feet like unto fine brass, as if they burned in a furnace; and his voice as the sound of many waters.*

The astral head is white like wool and is the thousand-petaled (rayed) super-electric lotus (main dynamo of life force) described in Yoga books. The origin of all concentrated finer forces which govern the physical body is in the head; hence the fine, hair-like filaments of white, fleecy lights in the main cerebral centre are described as white, fibrous and fluffy, *like wool.* The cerebral light of thousand petals or thousand rays, as described in Hindu Yoga books, performing the thousand-and-one functions in the body, is pure and *white as snow.* White is the combination of all colors; and the cerebral astral mother cell, the feeder of the above-mentioned seven life sub centres of different vibrations and colors, is described as *white.* The seven

13

subcentres manifest different colors, according to their rates of vibratory manifestations. *Different thoughts register different states and colors in the spiritual eye and life force.* The physical eyes proceed from one light centre, just as one switch lights the two headlights of an automobile. Thus the physical body has two eyes, but the astral body has only one eye, like *a flame of fire.* It is the one astral *flame of fire* which pours into the two eyes, giving them power and manifesting them as two. For this reason, when the two eye currents are concentrated and thrown back in the medulla by focusing the eyes on the point between the eyebrows, they are perceived as one single spiritual eye of light. (. . . *If therefore thine eye be single, thy whole body shall be full of light.*) When the two physical eyes manifest the single spiritual eye, then one can perceive, by continuous spiritual development, the physical body as filled with the super-lights of the supersensuous astral body. The astral head is pure white, the astral centres of lesser vibrations are golden, and the astral feet, with the lowest rate of vibration, glow yellow, like melted brass in a furnace.

Different thoughts change the life energy into different colors.

All vibratory manifestations are accompanied by lights or sounds, whether we register them or not; or rather, vibrations express themselves in us through various lights or sounds. The astral body consists of different rates of vibration, manifesting themselves in different colors and voices, or sounds of many waters, or vibrating elements. Different sounds emanate from the seven elements of the astral med-

14

ullary super-ether current, ether manifesting cervical current; air, or vitality, dorsal current; fire, lumbar current; water, sacral current, and the earth, coccygeal current. All these—super-ether in the medulla; ether in the cervical plexus; air current in the dorsal plexus; fire current in the lumbar plexus; water current in the sacral plexus, and earth current in the coccygeal plexus—are the different vibrating elements which constitute the human body, and they give forth different sounds. For this reason, this astral body of many lights and colors is spoken of as emanating from elements.

Different astral sounds and the Cosmic Sound (Aum or Om).

St. John heard the astral symphony and the one voice of many waters.

The astral body, besides manifesting the individual specific sounds from the seven different centres, also manifests the one *voice* as *the sound of many waters,* including both macrocosmic and microcosmic physical and astral elements. The Yogi, like St. John, can distinguish, by higher spiritual methods, the different sounds of the astral symphony, emanating from the coccygeal, sacral, lumbar, dorsal, cervical, and medullary plexuses,[1] respectively. Also the Yogi listens to the one Cosmic Voice or Sound of Om, ema-

[1]. *Medullary plexus* = Om Astral Symphony of all plexuses;
2. *Cervical plexus* = Roar of ocean;
3. *Dorsal plexus* = Long drawn out bell sound;
4. *Lumbar plexus* = Harp;
5. *Sacral plexus* = Flute;
6. *Coccygeal plexus* = Humming sound, like bumble-bee.

15

nating from *many waters* or elements, constituting the whole physical, astral, ideational macrocosmic and microcosmic universes. Hence, *the sound of many waters* spoken of by St. John is composed of the specific astral sounds of the seven plexuses and the one Cosmic Sound of Om. Both kinds of sounds are intuitively heard by the Yogi who has felt, or has had the vision of, the astral body.

Revelation 1:16   *And he had in his right hand seven stars: and out of his mouth went a sharp two-edged sword: and his countenance was as the sun shineth in his strength.*

Bliss-space, super-ether, ether.   Furthermore, the seven astral centres and their seven elements are manifested as seven stars of light. The seven elements, bliss-space (the super-fine medium in which bliss abides), super-ether (the fine semiconscious vibratory medium through which thoughts are transmitted), ether (the fine vibratory medium of energy), air, fire, water, and earth (of which the body is composed) are but the seven lotuses of life force or the seven frozen star-rayed currents. These seven stars, *burning in his right hand*

Astral cerebro-   in the proper channel of active force, or
spinal axis or   *Susumna,* or in the astral cerebrospinal
Susumna.   axis, remain as vibrating life currents feeding the seven elements, bliss-space, super-ether, ether, air, fire, water, and the earth elements in the body, keeping them constantly supplied and vibrating.

16

The conscious Cosmic Energy first enters through the medulla and remains concentrated in the brain as the thousand-petaled electric lotus. Then it descends into the body through spinal cord and the sympathetic nervous system. If these seven stars were extinguished and withdrawn from the proper channel of spinal vitality into the Spirit, the whole body would begin to decay. The body is frozen life current; therefore, as it decays under the influence of the heat of change, it must be kept frozen and fed by these constantly burning seven starry sentinels of life.

Medulla oblongata or mouth of God. We speak of the medulla as the *mouth of God* or the finite opening in the body of man through which God breathes His Cosmic Energy or Life into flesh. This medulla, also called the *mouth of the astral body,* emanates *a sharp two-edged sword,* or a powerful, two-edged, doubly serving positive-negative current. The one Cosmic Energy must create through the law of duality and relativity, so it sprouts forth the medullary seed current into two positive-negative currents. The birth of the two astral ganglia chains of the sympathetic system, the *Ida* current on the left and the *Pingala* current on

Ida and Pingala currents of astral sympathetic system. the right side of the spinal cord, is also made possible through the dual (two-edged) creative power of the medulla. The astral and the physical medulla are like two cloven half seeds of the positive-negative forces which give birth to the astral and physical nervous system. The astral medulla seed sprouts forth into

17

the vital tree of life, extending its pairs of branches into the two brain hemispheres, eyes, ears, hands, feet, as well as the two pairs of numerous inner organs. The two astral sympathetic nervous currents (*Ida* and *Pingala*) act in conjunction with the astral main central or spinal *Susumna* current. These two branches of life current emanate from the medulla seed and intertwine themselves with the *Susumna* vital current at the spinal centres. He who knows how to withdraw his life force from the body, muscles, and senses and draw it upwards through the spinal plexuses, opening the astral-physical knots of age-old attachment, can reach the cerebrum and behold the thousand-rayed energy lotus shining there in the astral countenance with the strength of thousand billions of crushed suns.

The light that Do you know why you experience
shineth behind darkness when you close your eyes?
the darkness. The gross light vibrations of the moon,
sun, and electricity blind your eyes to the powerful, mellow lights within. The average person's spiritual eye is closed but that of the Yogi is open, and he can see the inner lights at any time during the day or night. With the opening of the spiritual eye, a great light appears beyond the veil of darkness. That was St. John's meaning when he spoke of *the light that shineth behind the darkness.*

Revelation 1:17 *And when I saw him, I fell at his feet as dead. . . .*

St. John realized, like the Hindu Yogis, that when this

astral body is perceived as separate from the physical body, the energy being reversed to the Spirit, the physical body apparently consciously relaxes like that of a dead man. In conscious relaxation of the involuntary organs the astral energy goes out of the body, leaving it untenanted like a dark electric bulb from which the electricity has been switched off but can be switched on again at will. Then, beholding the separated astral body, one no longer perceives himself as a part of the perishable, brittle body bulb. When St. John *saw him,* or the astral body and Spirit above his head, he *fell at his feet as dead, i.e.,* he also perceived, in a conscious trance, his physical body, bereft of life force, lying at the feet or lower end of the floating astral body, apparently dead. Following the switched-off body current from the body bulb the soul perceives itself as an emanation of the immortal conscious Cosmic Ray which is the first Creator and the ultimate Absorber of all materialized objects. The Cosmic Ray is swallowing up all minor forms of energy, and the Cosmic Energy is being swallowed up by Conscious Space or Conscious Omnipresence. Then the soul realizes its immortality and is freed from the consciousness of physical death witnessed in many earthly incarnations. The delusion of death, born of the soul's identification with the body, is gone, and the soul perceives itself as alive forevermore.

These eternally true astral experiences were put in writing by St. John in order that flesh-identified brothers might find redemption from the consciousness of death, earthly changes, etc. One versed in the art of astrally separating the inner body from the physical body knows the causes of

19

mortal bondage, or hell. Such an one also knows how to open the doors of mortal change or death and escape into the kingdom of Changeless Infinity. *These*

The seven astral *eternal truths and seven astral doors of*
doors of escape. *escape from the prison of torturing*
matter are described by St. John to en-
able the awakened ones to fly to the home of Eternal Bliss.

Each *angel* occupies a *church;* each starry light occupies an astral *church* or *golden candlestick,* or one of the seven elements in the spine.

The experiences described by St. John can be realized by sincerely practicing the fourth and fifth Yogoda lessons, the Higher lesson on the Super-art of Realization, and the method given below.

A Yogi who can, as St. John, switch off the current from the body and listen to the Cosmic Vibration can, in an ad-vanced state, experience the *seven golden candlesticks* or seven astral doors of escape from the body to the Infinite.

Remember: Omnipresence was our throne. We became slaves, concentrating on the senses. We must return to Omnipresence. We are not only afraid of our omnipresence, but we even try to forget it. We must transfer the soul's attention from the changing, untrustworthy sense centres to the throne of Omnipresence. Sleep is the greatest messenger of Omnipresence. Every night the soul is given a chance to forget the little body and is enthroned in the vastness within.

It was the master's supreme wish that I pass these truths on to you; now it is "up to you" to apply them in every-day life. You have heard many lectures; what you need is study and practice in order to attain realization. The true spiritual way of studying scripture differs from the intellectual. Dozens of vague, meaningless books have been written on Revelation. Jesus Christ was crucified once, but His teachings are being crucified every day by misinterpretations. When you read this, meditate on it.

Heavenly Father! Transfer our consciousness from the physical body to the spine and from it through the seven centres to Cosmic Consciousness, where Thy glory and light reign in the fulness of Thy manifestation; where the Life Force reigns in all Thy power. Peace!

METHOD: Sit upright and straighten the spine to resemble a straight lightning rod. Concentrate the vision between the eyebrows with eyes half open. (Do not frown while doing this; keep the facial expression serene.) Now slightly move the spine to the left and right by swaying the body, changing the centre of your consciousness from the body and senses to the spine. Feel the astral spine and stop swaying the body. Then let your consciousness travel up and down several times, from the coccygeal plexus at the end of the spine to the point between the eyebrows. Then concentrate on the coccygeal plexus and mentally chant Om. Again, but slowly, travel up the spine, mentally feeling the coccygeal, sacral, lumbar, dorsal, cervical, and medullary plexuses, to the point between the eyebrows, mentally chanting Om in each place. When you reach the central point between the eyebrows, return downward, chanting Om at the point between the eyebrows, the medulla, and the five plexuses, and mentally feeling the centres at the same time. Continue to chant Om at the seven centres, feeling them while traveling up and down the astral spinal *Susumna* passage. Practice the above until you distinctly feel that your consciousness is transferred from the body into the spine.

The practice of the above method will release your soul from the bondage of matter and sense attachment by enabling you to escape through the seven astral doors and become one with the Spirit.

SUMMARY

The soul, having been encaged through ages in the three bodies—physical, astral, and ideational—is unable to cast off its shackles and escape into omnipresent Cosmic Consciousness.

The union of human consciousness with Cosmic Consciousness is impossible through imagination and intellectual study of the scriptural truths alone. Such union is possible only through knowledge of the above-mentioned seven astral spinal doors (the *seven golden candlesticks* and *stars*) and through withdrawing the life force and consciousness from the body into the Infinite and then bringing it back again. The soul, imprisoned in the body, must learn to free itself at will from its bondage. No matter what religion one professes, as he comes closer to real salvation, he is confronted with the necessity of opening the seven seals of energy and flesh in order to free the soul from the bondage of the body and unite it with the Spirit.

Both St. John in the Christian Bible and the Hindu savant Patanjali in his *Yoga Aphorisms* have spoken of this one scientific, psycho-spiritual seven-doored passage in the spine, through which all aspirants for salvation must pass to reach the Spirit consciously.

OUTLINE NOTES ON LESSON No. I

Q. What is Revelation? Ans. Revelation consists of those spiritual truths which were psycho-intuitively revealed to St. John and may be revealed to anyone with his state of super-consciousness.

God Consciousness transferred the spiritual truths to Jesus, the man with Christ Consciousness, who through his angel consciousness, or intuition, revealed them to his disciple John.

Revelation 1:2   *Who bare record . . . of all things that he saw.* All spiritual experiences were verified by the vibratory manifestation of God and the Christ Consciousness immanent in it.

Revelation 1:4   *. . . seven Spirits . . .* The seven manifestations of God also testified to the truth of St. John's spiritual experiences.

Revelation 1:5   *And from Jesus Christ, who is the*
Revelation 3:14   *faithful witness . . .* [See also *Revelation 3:14: . . . These things saith the Amen. the faithful and true witness, the beginning of the*

creation of God]; Jesus, the Christ Consciousness, and the Vibratory Word are the faithful witnesses of everything and the source of all power and grace (ordered creation). Consciousness and sound accompany all vibratory creation, just as the running of a motor is accompanied by a droning, humming sound. The intelligently working Cosmic Motor, planets, electrons, atoms—everything emanates the cosmic roar of Om. . . . *the first begotten of the dead* . . . [the Yogi's first contact with Christ Consciousness after he is dead, i.e., after he transcends the physical, astral, and ideational bodies by conscious meditation].

. . . *prince* . . . (supervisor) . . . *of the kings* . . . (forces of the earth or universe).

Revelation 1:8   *I am* . . . *the beginning and the ending* . . . (the vibratory relativity consisting of the beginning and end of all created things).

Revelation 1:9   . . . *word of God* . . . (vibratory manifestations of diverse true principles emanating from God).

Revelation 1:10   *I was in the Spirit* . . . [St. John's ego was contacting the Spirit, and he was not wholly allied with the physical consciousness].

. . . *on the Lord's day* . . . (on the day that the Lord revealed Himself as the Spirit—this can be any day for those who are spiritually awake).

. . . *heard behind me a great voice* . . . [spiritual vibration inaudible to human ears, hence intuitively perceived].

24

St. John was in the spiritual consciousness, hence he was free from the relativity of the dimensions and beyond the fourth dimension. Therefore, the word *behind* cannot mean direction but signifies that he was beyond the conscious and subconscious and in the superconscious state, and behind the gross bodily vibrations and the musical finer vibrations of the subtle body. *A great voice*—one great Cosmic Sound of Om emanating from Christ Consciousness and Cosmic Vibration or the Cosmic Motor. The word *voice* signifies vibration coming from a conscious Being. *As of a trumpet* —vibrations with variations. Hear the Om sound like the roar of the sea by the practice of the fifth Yogoda lesson. Om is the manifesting sound of intelligent Cosmic Vibration.

Revelation 1:11   *Saying* (declaring in the sound), *I am Alpha and Omega, the first and the last . . .* (The Om is the origin and end of everything. As motion causes the rise, momentary suspension, and dissolution of the wave, so the Cosmic Vibration of Om at a certain state creates, then preserves, and ultimately dissolves everything in the Infinite Sea).

Revelation 1:12   *And I turned to see the voice that spake with me . . .* [St. John *turned* his attention, to be one with *the voice* (conscious Cosmic Vibration) that was consciously vibrating within, suggesting infinite spiritual meanings]. *And being turned, I saw seven golden candlesticks;* [He saw, *i.e.,* intuitively felt, the seven receptacles (centres) of light- -not the lights themselves].

25

Revelation 1:13   And in the midst . . . one like unto
                      the Son of man . . . [Around the
seven centres as the base, he saw one subtle luminous body
like the physical body *(Son of man).*]

Revelation 1:14   His head and his hairs were white
                      like wool, . . . [The thousand-petaled
lotus of Life Energy is white and is the seat and origin of
all colors; wool suggests softness.] . . . *his eyes were as a
flame of fire*—(the third or spiritual eye burning as one
flame, and not the two gross flames of life energy which are
present in the physical two eyes).

Revelation 1:15   And his feet like unto fine brass . . .
                      [seat of grosser vibrations of lighter
color, as brass (yellow), symbolized as feet] . . . *and his
voice as the sound of many waters* (Christ Consciousness
and Cosmic Vibration manifested the varying Cosmic Sound
of Om).

Revelation 1:16   And he had in his right hand[1] seven
                      stars: . . . [His subtle body had in the
seat of stronger virtuous activity (the spine) seven condensed
luminous centres with seven different vibrations—the creators of the seven *tattwas* or elements.] . . . *and out of his
mouth went a sharp two-edged sword:* . . . [Out of the

[1]The right hand is the spine through which the Cosmic Current first descends,
with full power, into the body, and the left hand is the sympathetic nervous
system through which the life force flows comparatively more feebly.

26

luminous medulla proceeded two currents of optic life current which feed the two eyes and all other organs created in pairs.] . . . *and his countenance was as the sun shineth in his strength.* [The head is the seat of concentrated energy.]

Revelation 1:17   *And when I saw him, I fell at his feet as dead* . . . [During the time of the vision of the subtle body and the centres, there was relaxation of energy in the involuntary organs in the body; otherwise the outgoing life current would have kept the mind distracted with gross sensations. The death-like physical body was perceived in a conscious trance as resting under the hovering luminous feet of the astral body.]

Revelation 1:20   *Seven stars* . . . [the seven vibratory spiritually visible currents] . . . *seven golden candlesticks* . . . [seven centres or seats of the subtle energy star lotuses].

Super-Advanced Course No. 1

-•-❖-•-

Lesson No. 2

-•-❖-•-

DEVELOPING RESPONSE-BRINGING MENTAL WHISPERS: THE EASIEST AND SUREST METHOD OF ROUSING THE SPIRIT IN ANSWER TO YOUR DEMANDS.

By

SWAMI YOGANANDA

-•-❖-•-

This sacred lesson is meant only for the devoted Yogoda
student who would, untiringly and unceasingly,
seek God until he finds Him

-•-❖-•-

Published By
YOGODA SAT-SANGA SOCIETY
3880 San Rafael Avenue
Mount Washington
Los Angeles, Calif.

Your "needs" and Differentiate between your "needs"
your "wants." and your "wants." Your "needs" are
few, while your "wants" can be limit-
less. In order to find freedom and Bliss, minister only unto
your "needs"; stop creating limitless "wants" and pursuing
the will-o'-the-wisp of false happiness. The more you depend on conditions outside yourself for happiness, the less
happy you will be.

Fostering the desire for luxuries is the surest way to in-
creased misery. Don't be the slave of things or possessions;
boil down even your "needs." Spend your time in search
of lasting happiness or Bliss. The unchangeable, immortal
soul is hidden behind the screen of your consciousness on
which are painted dark pictures of disease, failure, death,
etc. Lift the veil of illusive change, and be established in
your immortal nature. Enthrone your fickle consciousness
on the changelessness and calmness within you, which is
the throne of God; then let your soul manifest Bliss night
and day.

Rise above the Beware! The mind must be protected
four mental from the four alternating psychological
states. states of sorrow, false happiness, indifference, and a deceptive, passive peace
which claims the ego for brief intervals, whenever it manages
to shake off the other three. Look at any face, and you will
be able to tell whether its owner is at the mercy of any one
of these. It is but rarely that people's faces remain calm
while they are in the grip of the four unstable mental states.

1

Whenever a desire for anything like health or pleasure is denied an individual, sorrow is born, which changes that person's face. "Prince Smile" is routed by "King Sadness" who tortures the muscles and distorts the expression.

Whenever a person's desire is fulfilled, he is temporarily "happy." Sorrow is born of unfulfilled desire; "happiness," of fulfilled desire. Sorrow and false happiness, like the Siamese Twins, dwell and travel together. They are the children of desire and are never far apart; if you invite "happiness," sorrow is sure to follow.

When the ego is not buffeted about by sorrow or "happiness," it sinks into the state of indifference. You can look around you and find the faces of many people register-ing this state of boredom.

You ask a person engrossed in indifference, "Are you sad?"

"Oh no," he replies.

Then you ask him, "Are you happy?"

"Oh no," he drawls.

"Well then," you ask, "what *is* the matter with you?"

"Oh," he cries, "I am just bored."

That is the mental state of many people.

Beyond these other changeable states, sorrow, false happi-ness, and indifference or mental inertia, lies the neutral state of passive mental peace. It is of a negative, short-lived nature—the aftermath of, and temporary lull in, the first-mentioned three states.

Beyond these four states of consciousness is the uncondi-tional, ever-new state of Bliss felt only in meditation.

2

How earthly   The soul, being individualized Spirit, *desires are born.*   if given a chance to unfold, can manifest all the fulfillment and satisfaction
of the Spirit. It is through long-continued contact with
changeable matter that material desires are developed.

Desire is an impostor which hampers, and encroaches
upon, your ever-joyous soul and lures your ego to dance
upon the crests of the four fluctuating, short-lived psychological states.

How to become   Protect the soul from the disturbance *a "Bliss billionaire."* created within your mind by the mad
dance of sorrow-producing desire.
Learn to overcome wild, wicked desire. Realize that you
do not need the things which create misery, for if you search
within your soul you will find there true happiness and lasting peace, or Bliss. Thus you will become a "Bliss billionaire."

What is true   The soul's nature is Bliss—a lasting *desirelessness?*   inner state of ever-new, ever-changing
joy, which eternally entertains without
changing the one entertained even when he passes through
the trials of physical suffering or death. Desirelessness is
not a negation; it is rather the attainment of the self-control
you need in order to regain your eternal heritage of all-
fulfillment lying within your soul. First give the soul the
opportunity to manifest this state, by Yogoda meditation,
and then, constantly living in this state, do your duty to

3

your body and mind and the world. You need not give up your ambitions and become negative; on the contrary, let the ever-lasting joy, which is your real nature, help you to realize all noble ambitions. Enjoy noble experiences with the Joy of God. Perform real duties with Divine Joy.

Play your tragic or comic parts in life with an inner smile. You are immortals, endowed with eternal joy. Never forget this during your play with changeable mortal life. This world is but a stage on which you play your parts under the direction of the Divine Stage Manager. Play them well, whether they be tragic or comic, always remembering that your *real* nature is eternal Bliss, and nothing else. The one thing which will never leave you, once you transcend the four unstable mental states, is the joy of your soul.

Therefore, learn to swim in the calm sea of unchanging Bliss before you attempt to plunge into the maelstrom of material life which is the realm of sorrow, pleasure, indifference, and a deceptive, temporary peace.

Proof of the existence of God as Bliss is felt in meditation. The whole-hearted practice of meditation as taught in the fifth Yogoda lesson brings deep Bliss. This ever-new Bliss is not born of desire; it manifests itself the moment the above-mentioned four mental states melt away by the magic command of your inner, intuition-born calmness. Manifest this serenity always. When Bliss comes over you, you will recognize it as a conscious, intelligent, universal Being to whom you may

4

appeal, and not as an abstract mental state. This is the surest proof that God is eternal, ever-conscious, ever-new Bliss.

How to make
your prayers
effective.
When you are experiencing this ever-new Bliss, never doubt that you are contacting God. It is at this time that your broadcasting microphone of prayer-demand is ready to transmit your mental whispers to Him.

Prayer vs.
demand.
Most people are absent-minded while they pray. Some love God but do not express that love continuously; hence their prayers are not answered. Moreover, a beggar supplicates; a child demands. A beggar's plea is of a fawning, groveling, cringing nature; a child's demand is straightforward, sincere, and lovingly unafraid. Most people *beg* from God; hence they receive a beggar's pittance instead of a son's share. Those who demand as children receive everything the Father has. A beggar *doubts* that his plea will be granted; a true son *knows* that his demand will be fulfilled. You *were* a son, but your own weakness has made you a beggar; you must become a son again before you can claim your birthright. Therefore, *demand to be a son again before you demand anything else. First establish your identity with God, as Jesus did, by realizing, in the, joy of meditation, "I and my Father are one."* Do not beseech Him beggarwise, but unite your ignorance-separated soul with God by constantly remaining identified with the ever-new Bliss within you.

5

Demand, after you have established your identity with God. After you have re-established your ever-new, joyous contact with Bliss-God, you may offer your demands for health, prosperity, or wisdom through mental whispers.

It is the purpose of this lesson to show the modern theology-blinded, theory-fed, belief-submerged human brother the way to contact God easily. To be able to do that, he must *know how to develop dynamic mental whispers.*

The world has done enough fruitless chanting and praying. Loud prayers are helpful in congregations if practiced with deep concentration and devotion; but, usually, when a person voices his prayers instead of mentally whispering them, they are said in "parrot fashion," while the mind is occupied with something else. God knows this; He does not answer when His name is taken in vain. Moreover, a voiced prayer absorbs the power of attention and is thus prevented from marching God-ward.

Contact God through inner mental whispers. *You know that whenever you want something very much, no matter what you may be doing, no matter where you may happen to be, a constant mentally whispering desire for the object forcibly rotates in the background of your mind. This haunting real desire for anything, I call a mental whisper.* The mind constantly whispers to itself what it wants. Such mental whisper bears no resemblance to parroted prayers; it is spontaneous and secretly works itself into a dynamic power.

6

An unceasing demand for anything, mentally whispered with unflinching zeal and unflagging courage and faith, develops into a dynamic power which so influences the entire behavior of conscious, subconscious, and superconscious powers of man, that the desired object is gained. A mental whisper, to achieve its object, must be undaunted by reverses and unceasing in its inner performance; then it will materialize.

Unknowingly, you have practiced such mental whispering many times, and have obtained results in the fulfillment of your desires.

Do away with the mockery of mechanical, loud praying. Shake off the false satisfaction of believing "just something" about God. You must *know* God. You must know how to rouse Him consciously and tangibly and make Him answer your demands. Do not rest until you have heard His voice *consciously*.

You can ease your conscience by claiming that pressure of business prevents you from praying and meditating, but you can have no excuses for not offering Him deep mental whispers at any time, in the temple of activity or on the altar of silence. No matter what you may be doing, you are always free to whisper your love to God, until you consciously receive His response. This is the surest way to contact Him in the mad rush of present-day life.

To rouse God, to receive His response, you must offer Him your mental-whisper songs unceasingly. No matter what you are doing, offer deep, inward mental-whisper prayer-demands with any of the following thoughts:

7

A few mental whispers. Make them your own by meditating on their meaning before offering them to God.

(1) Father, reveal Thyself.

(2) Beloved Divine Mother, hide no more. Blast the wall of ignorance, and appear unto me in all Thy splendor.

(3) Divine Mother, lift the veil of darkness which hangs before me whenever I meditate on Thee with closed eyes.

(4) Divine Mother, show Thyself in the light of my flaming love for Thee.

(5) Divine Friend, with my little arms I want to clasp Thy Omnipresence. Come! I can wait no more. Come!

(6) Beloved Spirit, burst through the opaque firmament of my selfishness-clouded love and embrace me with Thy omnipresent light.

(7) I will burn the door of silence with the fires of my ever-working dynamic inner whispers. O ever-burning Love, show Thyself in my flaming devotion.

(8) May the memory of Thy presence shine forever on the shrine of my whispering devotion. May my love for Thee burn secretly in the temple of Thy heart, and may I be able to awaken Thy love in all hearts.

(9) May Thy love burn forever on the altar of my heart, and may I be able to kindle love for Thee on all heart altars.

Thus, day by day, as you offer mental whispers, a new awakening will come; a new living relation with God will be established. The mist of silence and mystery, which hangs over everything, will slowly vanish before the dawning light of your mental whispers for God.

The blue sky will speak, saying, "Look! Here He is, spread all over my bosom." The flowers will say, "Behold His smile in us!" The dumb stones will declare, "See! He is sleeping in us." The trees will whisper, "He is dreaming in us." The birds will sing, "He is awake and singing in us." Your soul will say, "He is throbbing in me." Your hitherto unmindful, unconscious thoughts will say, "He is awake in thee now, awakened by thy inner whispers. Listen! Through thy soul-stirring whispers He is whispering songs of His love unto thee everywhere."

When your unceasing whispers shall at last dig deep into the soil of Omnipresent Silence, the fountains of His answering whispers will gush forth from your soul and with their life-giving waters refresh thirsting hearts everywhere.

SUMMARY

To receive God's response to your prayer-demands, ask only for that which you really need. The desire for superfluous material possessions ultimately brings misery and retards your spiritual progress.

Before demanding anything of God, first establish your identity with Him through meditation. Then demand, as a child of the Father, knowing that your request will be granted—not with the attitude of a beggar.

Many prayers are said absent-mindedly, consisting of empty words forced from without. When you meet a friend after a long absence, you do not consult books on friendship in order to know how to express your love to him. God is your closest Friend; let your prayer-demands to Him

9

be spontaneous outpourings, welling up from the depths of your heart.

Whenever you have a real need, the thought of it is in your mind all the time, no matter where you are or what you are doing. Developing such deep, dynamic, inner whispers is sure to bring a response from Him. Constantly, unceasingly, whisper unto Him of your eternal love, of your burning desire to contact Him.

"Offer deep mental whispers in the temple of scientific meditation until you hear His answering whispers every-where, audibly and distinctly."

Super-Advanced Course No. 1

-.+.-

Lesson No. 3

-.+.-

REVERSING THE SEARCHLIGHTS OF THE SENSES.
WHERE IS YOUR CONSCIOUSNESS CENTRED?
IN WHAT SLUMS IS YOUR SOUL ROAMING?

By

SWAMI YOGANANDA

-.+.-

This sacred lesson is meant only for the devoted Yogoda
student who would, untiringly and unceasingly,
seek God until he finds Him

-.+.-

Published By
YOGODA SAT-SANGA SOCIETY
3880 San Rafael Avenue
Mount Washington
Los Angeles, Calif.

What is the ego? The soul's subjective consciousness of the body and its other material relations is termed the ego. The soul itself, being individualized Spirit, should manifest only its kinship with the Spirit, which is unmanifested, ever-existing, ever-conscious, ever-new Bliss. Hence, as Its reflection the soul, in its true state, is individualized, ever-existing, ever-conscious, ever-new Bliss. The ego, however, being identified with the three bodies—ideational, astral, and physical—(and their normal-abnormal conditions), has put on their natures.

Watching the wanderings of the ego. It is extremely necessary for the advanced student on the path of meditation to *watch the wanderings of his ego in the realms of consciousness*—in other words, the wanderings of "King Soul" in the form of matter-stricken ego.

The physical, astral, and ideational planes must all be comprehended through consciousness. Therefore, we can safely say that when we are in an undeveloped state the roamings of the ego in the "Kingdom of Consciousness" interest us only during the twenty-four man-made terrestrial hours.

The human ego generally travels in the realm of sensation during the waking state. After the curtain of dreams is drawn, the ego semiconsciously roams in the chamber of dreams. It may be said to be semiconscious while dreaming,

1

because it dimly perceives the dream pictures during their performance and can recall them after waking.

Human con-
sciousness is
never wholly
suspended.
During the dream state, the ego is semi-unconscious of the world and of sense experiences—yet it is conscious of the dream world. It is also conscious of deep sleep while in that state. The link between consciousness and subconsciousness is unbroken; otherwise dreams could not be recalled when consciousness is fully resumed. It is impossible to be wholly unconscious; the soul's subjective consciousness, or the ego, may be asleep or resting, but this can never be termed "unconsciousness."

During retirement to the subconscious dream chamber, consciousness casts off its garment of the gross sensations of touch, smell, taste, sight, and audition. But though divested of its physical sense instruments of perception, consciousness still retains its intuitive powers of cognition through the subconscious, and beholds the dreams resulting from memories, thoughts, and the activity of the subtle senses, the mental reflexes of the physical senses. (For instance, nearly every one can recall vivid dreams of eating ice cream, hot pie, or other foods.) However, when the ego enters the silent chamber of deep sleep or semi-superconsciousness, its experiences consist of the unalloyed enjoyment of real peace. The human consciousness, turned within, here begins to resume

2

its normal state of calmness, peace, and joy. The conscious state is marked by restlessness; the subconscious state, by a mixture of restfulness and activity, but Bliss reigns in the superconscious state.[1]

The ego is peaceful in the realm of semi-superconsciousness, subtly excited or pleased in the dream state, and grossly excited or pleased while experiencing gross sensations.

The links of consciousness. Ordinarily, during its stay in the chamber of sensations, while in the state of physical consciousness, the ego is linked with subconsciousness through memory and with superconsciousness through the sense of inward peace—manifested or unmanifested.

Determine which "throne" of consciousness your ego occupies, i. e., which consciousness is predominant in your mind.

Determining and changing the predominant state of consciousness. During waking hours, the conscious state is predominant, the subconscious and superconscious states trailing behind. By the power of concentration, you can make the subconscious or superconscious predominant. The conscious state of restlessness can

[1]The three states of consciousness and the physical and mental reactions produced by them:
1. Consciousness=Restlessness.
2. Subconsciousness=Restfulness and activity.
3. Semi-superconsciousness=Negative peace.
   Superconsciousness=Positive peace or Bliss.

be changed into the dreamy state of subconsciousness or the supremely peaceful state of superconsciousness. *In poets, the subconscious usually predominates; in business men, the conscious state, and in real Yogis and great Swamis, the superconscious state. Change your centre from conscious to superconscious predominance.*

The average man generally concentrates, and stays, on the plane of physical consciousness. But when he is forcibly (through drugs) or passively (through fatigue) led to the subconscious chamber of dreams and quiet sleep, or when he enters the semi-superconsciousness of joyous sleep, his ego generally becomes apparently unconscious or dimly conscious. The ordinary ego can support only one state at a time: the physically conscious state, or the subconscious state, or the semi-superconscious state.

In the untrained ego, sidetracked on the path of upward evolution, the conscious state always predominates. It loves to stay and dream in, and be conscious of, the realm of the senses only. It forgets that during the night it moves semi-consciously through the chamber of dreams or through deep semi-superconscious sleep toward the Spirit.

Consciousness is manifested through gross sensation; subtle astral subconsciousness is manifested through dreams, quiet negative sleep, and through memory which never sleeps.

This subconscious mind is always awake; it works through memory while consciousness predominates, runs the motion-picture theatre of dreamland, and enjoys serenity during negative sleep.

4

Business man   Consciousness, subconsciousness, and
vs. Yogi.   superconsciousness are different degrees
or states of Christ Consciousness—they
can never be entirely independent of one another, although
one state is usually stronger than the others. The ordinary
man works with consciousness predominating; in the Yogi
superconsciousness predominates. *Ask yourself at different
times during the day which consciousness is predominant
in you.*

Business men, in whom, as a rule, the conscious state predominates, as well as those who stay on the subconscious
plane, are unbalanced and one-sided, their happiness depending upon the circumstances in which they find themselves.
The superconscious individual is not enslaved by conditions
outside of himself; he is free and finds happiness within in
spite of all circumstances.

The mind can   The close relation between body and
control the body.   mind causes a psychological state to be
followed by a corresponding physio-
logical reaction which, in turn, intensifies the psychological
state. Be angry and your face will show it. Permit anger to
spread through your muscles until you are tense all over, and
your anger will increase. The Yogi, by adopting certain
psychological states, can produce the corresponding physio-
logical reactions, and vice versa, and by certain physical acts
he can instantaneously produce the corresponding psycho-

logical states. For instance, during sleep the eyes are closed; so by closing the eyes, the Yogi can produce instantaneous sleep at any time, anywhere. During the waking state the eyes are open—generally leveled; hence, by keeping the eyes level, the Yogi can remain consciously awake for days and weeks. Moreover, during the superconscious state and in death, when the soul races toward the superconscious, the eyes automatically go upward; so by lifting his eyes upward and focusing his vision on the point between the eyebrows, the Yogi can switch off the motion pictures of dreams or sensations at will and launch into the sea of luminosity, where electrons and life forces and Bliss reign in the "Kingdom of Spirit."

Becoming king of Meditation is the conscious method of
three kingdoms. entering the subconscious and superconscious realms. By learning to control your eye muscles and shifting the gaze at will, you can transfer your ego from the conscious world to the tranquillity of the subconscious dream world or to the superconscious state of perfect joy. Think of the freedom you gain by learning to shift, at will, from the land of terrestrial horror to the land of beautiful dreams, and when even dream fairies bother you, to float in the ether of eternal serenity or Bliss where dreams dare not tread or disturb. You are the king of three kingdoms. Realize that. Do not remain imprisoned in, and identified with, the little island of the body.

6

The Yogi has
complete control
over all forms
of consciousness.
The Yogi can do just as he pleases— he can live in the realm of the senses, or fly to the land of dreams, or float in the vast ocean of eternal Bliss. He may choose superconscious serenity or sub-conscious dreams; or he may give predominance to semi-superconsciousness, superconsciousness, or Christ Consciousness, at will. If he prefers, he may remain half conscious and half dreaming, or half conscious and half asleep yet dreamless, or he may be semi-superconscious and half dreaming or quietly subconscious. If none of these pleases him, he may elect to enjoy, simultaneously, conscious sensations, dreams, tranquillity, subconsciousness, semi-superconsciousness, superconsciousness, and immanent Christ Consciousness. When he can do that, his ego becomes soul, and his soul breaks its bubble walls and becomes the sea of Spirit— then it attains the state of *Nirbikalpa Samadhi* or transcendental Cosmic Consciousness. In this state he perceives that his "throne" of consciousness rests in the Omnipresent Heart of consciousness, subconsciousness, dream subconsciousness, semi-superconsciousness, superconsciousness, immanent Christ Consciousness, and transcendental Cosmic Consciousness, equally and co-existently, all the time.[1] Then

[1]Traveling by automobile, while on the plane of Cosmic Consciousness, often all at once I perceive co-existing in me, in infinite harmony, the car and the scenery surrounding it; my thoughts; my dreams; tranquillity; planets; the inner world of many-colored lights; my glistening feelings; intuition—in short, all forms of consciousness—playing their part in the Cosmic Symphony. My soul has merged into the Infinite, and I perceive my body as a tiny, hardly visible moth of light.

the "throne" of consciousness, instead of resting on a little speck of sensation, or a "diamond-chip" dream, or a little shining ambition, becomes fixed in the sparkling bosom of Omnipresence.

Technique for producing different states of consciousness. Relax your body in a sitting posture. Lean against the back of a comfortable chair. Close your eyes and forget your worries, dismissing all restless thoughts; feel drowsy, become passive and mentally "careless"; in other words, "let go," fall asleep, or at least try to doze. Repeat this several times until the minute you lower the searchlight of your vision, the eyes, closing them and switching off the optical currents, you are instantly submerged in the subconscious.

Then, whenever you are heavy with sleep, quickly tense the whole body and lift your drooping eyes, leveling them in front of you. Keep looking at one object without winking; banish sleep at will. Then close your eyes, relax, and fall asleep again.

Every night, before dropping off to sleep, command your subconscious mind to wake you at a different hour. Continue making this suggestion to the subconscious mind until it obeys. Fall asleep with the thought that a matter of vital importance depends upon your getting up at your appointed hour.

After you have trained your subconscious mind to waken you at will, practice fixing your vision on the point between the eyebrows, and instantaneously go consciously into the

8

state of deep peace, of deep intoxicating joy. The regular practice of the fourth and fifth Yogoda lessons and the higher methods will help you to attain this.

Empty your mind of thoughts. Every time thoughts return, firmly dismiss them. Then meditate on peace; be drunk with it; merge in it; consciously sleep over it.

Remember, to gain dominion over the three kingdoms, you must practice these exercises all the time. Whenever you have a period of leisure, lower and close your eyes and enter the "Kingdom of Dreams" at will. Then return at will, leveling your eyes, and enter the "Kingdom of Consciousness," drinking in the beauties of nature. Then lift your vision up between the eyebrows and enter the superconscious "Kingdom of Bliss."

You can attain complete freedom from worldly cares only after you have learned to shift the searchlight of your attention and energy from the conscious to the subconscious plane, or from the conscious to the superconscious plane, either dreaming or enjoying Bliss at will. *Then you can fly from the plane of sensations to the plane of dreams or to the realm of eternal peace, as you choose.*

Remember, however, that as you shift your vision from the conscious to the subconscious, the life force and energy must also be switched off from the lamps of the billion-celled muscles and the visual, auditory, olfactory, tactual, and gustatory nerves.

In shifting from the conscious to the superconscious plane, your lungs must be breathless, your heart calm, your cells inactive, your circulation stilled, and you must be listening to the symphony of the Cosmic Vibration of Om.

While in the superconscious state, one experiences complete *cessation* of unrest—*fruition* of peace—*soul-expansion,* unhampered by the friction attending sensations in the realm of consciousness.

If anyone claimed that he could sleep while he was running, he would be ridiculed, for healthful sleep is always accompanied by sensory and motor relaxation. Many profess to have attained Cosmic Consciousness, who have not yet learned to relax at will. The first signs of the attainment of Cosmic Consciousness are the fixed gaze, the consciously stilled heart, and breathlessness. If one cannot demonstrate these, he has not attained Cosmic Consciousness.

Contacting inner entities. After you have learned to do this at will, you may practise the following exercise, at night: Lean against the back of a chair. Close your eyes and shift your gaze from the conscious level downward to the subconscious level and fall asleep. Then invoke the souls which have passed on, and meet them there in your consciously arranged reception-parlor of dreamland.

To invoke Christ-like superconscious souls, however, you must extend a superconscious invitation. Lift your gaze and fix it between the eyebrows. Float away to the region of Bliss. In the chamber of Infinity and Perennial Peace in-

10

voke superconscious souls; they will come to you, materializing themselves from the Cosmic Consciousness into distinct saintly forms. The saints who became one with Spirit can be recreated by the Spirit. The Spirit Sea becomes a bubble of saintly life. Then, when this bubble of life knows itself as the Cosmic Sea, it merges with It. The Spirit Sea can reassume any form which It has once occupied and manifested. The Spirit is ever conscious. It has an eternal, unfailing memory. These superconscious souls sometimes descend from the Cosmic Consciousness, taking various forms of light, as the *Devas,* so that they might float about the astral spheres of million-hued mellow, spiritual lights, worshipping God in the land of super-electrons and love, and after entertaining Him with the astral "super-talkies" they return to the sphere of Cosmic Consciousness and vanish in the one Infinite Love.

High spiritual development increases one's capacity for enjoyment. Color becomes more brilliant, sound more marvelous, feeling more intense the farther one advances along the spiritual path.

Liberate "King Soul" from his bondage to body matter, the senses, and other attachments; lift his searchlight (attention) upward, from petty things to Infinity; from worldly pleasures to Eternal Joy; from the little body to the Universe; from the limited human consciousness to Cosmic Consciousness.

The little searchlight of attention and the five senses ordinarily are focused on imperfect matter. When thrown

11

back upon the Spirit, they disclose the Infinite Perfect Light forever dancing on God's fountain of Bliss, eternally emanating from Omnipresence and Christ Consciousness.

SUMMARY

Man's attachment to matter keeps the soul confined to the body prison and prevents it from finding freedom with God in the realm of Eternal Bliss. The ego attempts to satisfy the soul's constant, insatiable longing for God through material channels. Far from accomplishing its objective, it increases man's misery. *The soul's hunger can never be appeased by indulgence of the senses.* When man realizes this and masters his ego, *i.e.,* when he achieves *self-control,* life becomes glorified by Bliss while he is still in the flesh. Then, instead of being the slave of material desires and appetites, his attention is transferred to the heart of Omnipresence, resting there forever with the hidden Joy in everything.

Super-Advanced Course No. 1

--*-*

Lesson No. 4

--*-*

ART OF FINDING TRUE FRIENDS OF
PAST INCARNATIONS
WHAT IS FRIENDSHIP?

By

SWAMI YOGANANDA

--*-*

This sacred lesson is meant only for the devoted Yogoda
student who would, untiringly and unceasingly,
seek God until he finds Him

--*-*

Published By
YOGODA SAT-SANGA SOCIETY
3880 San Rafael Avenue
Mount Washington
Los Angeles, Calif.

What is friendship? Friendship is the universal spiritual attraction which unites souls in the bond of divine love and may manifest itself either in two or in many. The Spirit was One; by the law of duality it became two—positive and negative. Then, by the law of infinity applied to the law of relativity, it became many. Now the One in the many is endeavoring to unite the many and make them One. This effort of the Spirit to unify many souls into the One works through our emotions, intelligence, and intuition and finds expression through friendship.

To have friends, you must manifest friendliness. If you open the door to the magnetic power of friendship, a soul or souls of like vibrations will be attracted to you. The more friendly you become toward all, the greater will be the number of your real friends. *Friendship is a manifestation of God's love for you, expressed through your friends.*

Friendship and Cosmic Consciousness. There are people who do not trust anyone, and who utterly doubt the possibility of ever having true friends. Some, in fact, actually boast that they get along without friends. If you fail to be friendly, you disregard the divine law of self-expansion, by which alone your soul can grow into the Spirit. No man who fails to inspire confidence in other hearts—who is unable to extend the kingdom of his love and friendliness into other soul territories—can hope to spread his consciousness over Cosmic Consciousness. If you cannot conquer human hearts, you cannot conquer the Cosmic Heart.

1

Avoid doing anything which brings harm to yourself or to another. If you are self-indulgent, or if you encourage a friend in his vices, you are an enemy disguised as a friend. By being your own and others' true friend, you gain the friendship of God. Once you make your love felt in others' love, it will expand until it becomes the one Love which flows through all hearts.

Selfish attachment is the canker of friendship. True friendship is broad and inclusive. Selfish attachment to a single individual, excluding all others, inhibits the development of Divine Friendship. Extend the boundaries of the glowing kingdom of your love, gradually including within them your family, your neighbors, your community, your country, all countries—in short, all living sentient creatures. Be also a cosmic friend, imbued with kindness and affection for all of God's creation, scattering love everywhere. Such was the example set by Christ, Swami Shankara, and my masters (Babaji, Lahiri Mahasaya, and Swami Sriyukteswarji).

Realize your kinship with all mankind. *Consider no one a stranger; learn to feel that everybody is your kin.* Family love is merely one of the first exercises in the divine Teacher's course in Friendliness, intended to prepare your heart for an all-inclusive love. Feel that the life blood of God is circulating in the veins of all races. How does anyone dare to hate any human being

2

of whatsoever race when he knows that God lives and breathes in all? We are Americans or Hindus, etc., for just a few years, but we are God's children forever. The soul cannot be confined within man-made boundaries; its nationality is Spirit; its country, Omnipresence.

This does not mean that you must know and love all human beings and creatures *personally and individually*. All you need do is to be ready at all times to spread the light of friendly service over all living creatures which you happen to contact. This requires constant mental effort and preparedness; in other words, unselfishness. The sun shines equally on diamond and charcoal, but the one has developed qualities which enable it to reflect the sunlight brilliantly, while the other absorbs it all. Emulate the diamond in your dealings with people; brightly reflect the light of God's love.

All this may seem very complicated, but when you touch the Infinite, your difficulties will melt away. Divine Love will come to you; beautiful intuitive experiences of universal friendliness will play like fountains in your mind.

Constant contact with the Infinite in meditation fills one with Divine Love, which alone enables him to love his enemies

Why love your enemies? The secret of Christ's strength lay in His love for all, even His enemies. Far better to conquer by love the heart of a person who hates you than to vanquish him by other means. To the ordinary man such a doctrine seems absurd. He

3

wants to return ten slaps for the one he has received and add twice as many kicks for good measure. Why should you love your enemy? In order that you may bring the healing rays of your love into his dark, hatred-stricken heart. When it is so released, it can behold itself as pure golden love. Thus will the flame of your love burn the partitions of hatred and misery which separate your soul from other souls and all souls from the vast sea of Infinite Love.

How to convert enemies into friends. Practice loving those who do not love you. Feel for those who do not feel for you. Be generous to those who are generous only to themselves. If you heap hatred on your enemy, neither he nor you are able to perceive the inherent beauty of your soul.

You need not fawn on your enemy. Silently love him. Silently be of service to him whenever he is in need, *for love is real only when it is useful and expresses itself through action.* Thus will you rend the veils of hate and of narrow-mindedness which hide God from your sight.

If humility and apologies on your part bring out your enemy's good qualities, by all means apologize. The person who can do this will have attained a definite spiritual development, for it takes character to be able to apologize graciously and sincerely. It is the consciousness of his own inferiority which makes a man hide behind a display of pride. *Do not, however, encourage a wrongdoer by being humble and apologetic.*

4

Service is the
keynote of
friendship.
Cultivate true friendliness, for only thus do you attract true friends to your-self. True friendship consists in being mutually useful; in offering your friends good cheer in distress, sympathy in sorrow, advice in trouble, and material help in times of real need. Friendship consists in rejoicing in your friends' good fortune and sympathizing with them in adversity. Friendship gladly forgoes selfish pleasures or self-interest for the sake of a friend's happiness, without consciousness of loss or sacrifice; without counting the cost.

Never be sarcastic to a friend. Do not flatter him unless it be to encourage him; do not agree with him when he is wrong. Real friendship cannot witness with indifference the false, harmful pleasures of a friend. This does not mean that you must quarrel. Suggest mentally, or if your advice is asked, give it gently and lovingly. Fools fight; friends discuss their differences.

Help your friend also by being a mental, esthetic, and spiritual inspiration to him.

Friendship should not be influenced by people's relative positions. Friendship may and should exist between lovers, employer and employe, teacher and pupil, parents and chil-dren, and so forth.

Unfailing laws of
friendship.
Be neither unduly familiar with, nor indifferent to, a friend. Moreover, do not trade-mark him by telling him, "I know all about you." Respect and love grow among friends

5

with time. "Familiarity breeds contempt" between those who are mutually useless, selfish, materially minded, and unproductive of inspiration or self-development. The greater the mutual service, the deeper the friendship. Why does Jesus have such a wide following? Because He, like the other great masters, is unequaled in His service to humanity. Hence, to attract friends, you must possess the qualities of a real friend. Idiots may become friends, but their blind friendship may end in a sudden blind hate. The building of wisdom and spiritual and intuitive understanding by mutual effort alone can bind two souls by the laws of everlasting, universal Divine Love. Human love and friendship have their basis in service on the physical, mental, or business plane; they are short-lived and conditional. Divine Love has had its foundation in service on the spiritual and intuitional planes and is unconditional and everlasting.

How to achieve   *Unless conjugal love has a spiritual* *conjugal happiness. basis it can never last.* If husbands and wives are to live in friendship and harmony, they must be of spiritual service to each other. It is the "newlyweds" who forget that true (spiritual) love is based on unselfish mutual service and friendship, who soon come to a parting of the ways. When two souls are ideally mated, their love becomes spiritualized and is registered in eternity after death as the one love of God.

Finding friends of   There are people with whom you *past incarnations.* come in daily contact, yet with whom you do not feel in sympathy. Learn to love them and adapt yourself to them. There are others who

6

give you the instantaneous feeling that you have known them always. *This indicates that they are your friends of previous incarnations.* Do not neglect them, but strengthen the friendship existing between you. Be on the lookout for them always, as your restless mind may fail to recognize them. Often they are very near you, drawn by the friend-ship born in the dim, distant past. They constitute your shining collection of soul jewels; add to it constantly. In these bright soul galaxies you will behold the one Great Friend smiling at you radiantly and clearly. It is God who comes to you in the guise of a noble, true Friend, to serve, inspire, and guide you.

Ugliness of disposition and selfishness drive away all friends of former incarnations, whereas friendliness draws them toward you. Therefore, be ready always to meet them halfway. Never mind if one or two friends prove false and deceive you.

Each individual has his own standard of physical and mental beauty. What seems ugly to one may appear beauti-ful to another. *Looking at a vast crowd, you like some faces instantaneously; others do not attract you particularly.* The instant attraction of your mind to the likeable inner and outer features of an individual is your first indication that you have found a friend of the past. Your dear ones whom you loved before, will be drawn toward you by a prenatal sense of friendship.

Do not be deceived by physical beauty; ask yourself whether or not a face, the manner of walking—in short, everything about a person—appeals to you. Sometimes

7

overeating and lack of exercise may distort the features of a friend, and thus he may escape your recognition. Sometimes a beautiful woman may fall in love with an ugly man, or a handsome man, with a physically unattractive woman, due to the loving friendship of a past incarnation. A fat, distorted body may harbor a real friend. Therefore, to be sure that your eyes have not deceived you regarding the physical characteristics of your supposed former friend, ascertain whether you are mentally and spiritually congenial. Delve deeply into a person's mind and guard yourself against being prejudiced by little peculiarities, in order to find out whether your tastes and inclinations essentially agree. *Seek your friends of past incarnations in order that you may continue your friendship in this life and perfect it into Divine Friendship. One lifetime is not always sufficient to achieve such perfection.*

Jealousy is self-love and the death of friendship.

The ennobling effects of friendship. When true friendship exists between two souls and they seek spiritual love and God's love together, when their only wish is to be of service to each other, their friendship produces the flame of the Spirit. Through perfected Divine Friendship, mutually seeking spiritual perfection, you will find the one Great Friend.

When perfect friendship exists either between two hearts or within a group of hearts in a spiritual organization, such friendship perfects each individual. In the heart, purified by friendship, one beholds an open door of unity through

8

which he should invite other souls to enter—those that love him as well as those that love him not.

Friendship is God's love shining through the eyes of your loved ones, calling you home to drink His nectar of all differences-and-selfishness-dissolving unity. Friendship is God's trumpet call, bidding the soul to destroy the partitions which separate it from all other souls and from Him. True friendship unites two souls so completely that they reflect the unity of Spirit and Its divine qualities.

When you behold, assembled all at once beneath the canopy of your perfected universal friendship, the souls of the past, present, and future, the busy stars, the amœba, the whippoorwill, the nightingale, the dumb stones, and the shining sea sands, then the friendship thirst of your heart will be quenched forever. Then God's creation will ring with the emancipating song of all difference-dissolving celestial friendship. Then the Divine Friend will rejoice to see you come home after your evolutional wanderings and roamings through the pathways of incarnations. Then He and you will merge in the Bliss of Eternal Friendship.

Heavenly Father! Let those that are our own come unto us, and finding them may we find friendship with all, and thus find Thee.

SUMMARY

God's effort to unite strife-torn humanity manifests itself within your heart as the friendship instinct.

Make every effort to rediscover your friends of past incarnations, whom you may recognize through familiar physical, mental and spiritual qualities. Rising above considerations of material or even spiritual gain, perfect your friendship, begun in a preceding incarnation, into Divine Friendship.

When Divine Friendship reigns supreme in the temple of your heart, your soul will merge with the vast Cosmic Soul, leaving far behind the confining bonds which separated it from all of God's animate and inanimate creation.

Super-Advanced Course No. 1

--+--

Lesson No. 5

--+--

THE DIVINE MAGNETIC DIET: PHYSICAL AND MENTAL METHODS FOR REJUVENATING THE BODY CELLS AND AWAKENING THE LATENT POWERS OF THE MIND AND THE INNER FORCES OF THE SOUL

By

SWAMI YOGANANDA

--+--

This sacred lesson is meant only for the devoted Yogoda
student who would, untiringly and unceasingly,
seek God until he finds Him

--+--

Published By
YOGODA SAT-SANGA SOCIETY
3880 San Rafael Avenue
Mount Washington
Los Angeles, Calif.

Most diseases can be cured by judicious fasting under the guidance of a specialist.

Fasting may be divided into two main groups: *partial fasting* and *complete fasting*.

Partial Fasting: In this group, four general subdivisions may be mentioned:
- (I)   Limiting the diet to certain foods;
- (II)   Abstaining from certain foods;
- (III) Limiting the food intake as to quantity;
- (IV)   Limiting the number of meals to one or two per day.

Some of these forms of fasting may be combined. For instance, to cure disease or reduce weight, a person may abstain from certain foods altogether and limit the intake of other foods, etc.

More specific subdivisions are:

Liquid diet: (a) "Liquid" fasting. For one or two days a week, and whenever one does not feel hungry, the food intake may be confined to (1) milk, or (2) orange juice or any other fruit juice.

Solid diet: (b) "Solid" fasting. This diet is confined to (1) raw fruits;[1] (2) raw vegetables;[1] (3) half-boiled vegetables, including juice in which they were boiled.[1] Drink plenty of water while on this diet.

[1]No bread or other starchy foods or sugar; no meat, eggs, or fish—nothing but the foods mentioned in (1) or (2) or (3), and only one meal per day (at noon).

"Oxygen" diet: (c) "Oxygen" fasting. Inhaling and exhaling deeply from six to twelve times every hour, filling the lungs with fresh air down to the lower lobes. This method may be practiced outdoors for twelve hours, while alternately slowly walking and resting. When weather conditions necessitate indoor practice, the windows should be kept wide open. (Of course, warm clothing should be worn during the winter season as a protection against the cold.) This fast aids spiritual growth. It should not be undertaken by weak individuals or invalids.

Complete Fasting: Complete fasting should not, as a rule, exceed ten days and should not be attempted even for that length of time except under the supervision of a specialist. However, abstaining from food for one day each week and for three consecutive days each month, has brought beneficial results. Water must be taken in abundance during complete fasting, to replace the fluid lost by evaporation through the pores, etc.

Nine-day diet: The *Nine-day Cleansing and Vitalizing Diet,* given below, has proved a most effective method for ridding the system of poisons.

1½ grapefruit
1½ lemons, 5 oranges
1 cooked vegetable w i t h juice (quantity optional)
1 raw vegetable salad

1 glass orange juice with tsp.[1] Senna Leaves or new Original Swiss Kriss[2]
3 cups vitality beverage (one at each meal)

[1]tsp. = teaspoonful.
[2]To be taken every night while on cleansing diet, before going to bed. To obtain best results, take ½ tsp. at first; later increase to 1 tsp. Note that for invalids and children one should use proper care and discretion in going on this cleansing diet, and if necessary consult a specialist first.

2

Vitality Beverage: Ingredients for beverage:

2 stalks chopped celery	1/2 qt.[1] chopped dandelion
5 carrots (chopped) incl. part of stem	or turnip greens or spinach
1 bunch chopped parsley	1 qt. water

No salt or spices

The beverage may be prepared in two ways, the first being preferable:

(1) After putting celery and carrots through meat chop-per, lightly boil them in the water for ten minutes. Then add selected greens and parsley and boil ten minutes more. Strain by squeezing through cheesecloth.

(2) Use the same ingredients, but do not cook them. After putting them through meat chopper, strain as above. Drink one cup of the beverage, prepared by either method, at each of the three meals.

This vitality beverage has been found to be a blood tonic and very effective in rheumatism, various stomach disorders (including acute indigestion), chronic catarrh, bronchitis, and nervous "breakdown."

While on the cleansing diet, strictly abstain from spices, candies, pastries, meat, eggs, fish, cheese, milk, butter, bread, fried foods, oil, beans—in fact, all other foods not mentioned above. If one feels the need of additional nourishment, one may take a tablespoonful of thoroughly ground nuts in a half glass of water or a glass of orange juice.

[1]qt. = quart.

3

Following the nine-day diet, one should be especially careful in the selection and quantity of one's food intake the first day and resume a normal diet gradually.

If one is not successful in ridding the body of *all* poisons during the initial attempt, the cleansing diet may be repeated after an interval of two or three weeks.

While on the cleansing diet, it has been found beneficial every night just before going to bed, to use two pounds of some good bath salts in one-fourth tub of warm water; and also very helpful to take a bath salts bath every now and then, for several weeks after finishing the cleansing diet.

Reducing diet: One should Practice Exercise B of Yogoda Lesson 1 (recharging exercise), six times, twice a day, and exercises D and E of the same lesson (stomach exercises), twenty times each, three times a day. Command your will, during tension, to burn up the superfluous tissues. Practice the running exercise 50 to 200 times a day. Eat mostly raw vegetables and one-half of a boiled yolk of an egg a day. Abstain from starchy food, fried foods, and sweets. Do not drink water with meals. Every three days fast one day on orange juice.

Extremely stout people have derived much benefit from *fasting on orange juice seven days and then going on the nine-day cleansing diet, a normal diet being resumed gradually thereafter. If there was need for further reduction of weight, this procedure was repeated after an interval of two weeks.*

4

"Fattening" diet: The following foods are of high nu-
tritive value and have been found bene-
ficial for those who wish to gain weight:

bananas with cream	2 eggs
oatmeal with cream	1 large raw vegetable salad
1/4 glass cream	1 tbsp.[1] olive oil
2 slices whole-wheat bread	3 1/2 oz. butter

Weight has also been gained by eating bananas in abundance, and for one month drinking two glasses of water
(moderately hot or cold, *not iced*) with each meal.

Some of the foods from the above list are added to the
usual dietary.

General dietary   To have faith in God's healing power
rules: through the mind and obey dietary laws,
                              is better than just to have faith in God
and mind and disregard dietary laws.

Every day, for beneficial results, eat green-leafed vegetables, including a carrot with part of its stem, and drink a
glass of orange juice (including pulp) with a tablespoonful
of finely ground nuts. Mix good salad dressings made of
thoroughly ground nuts, cream, a few drops of lemon juice,
orange juice and honey with all salads. Thousand-island
dressing is good. A little curry sauce with boiled egg or
vegetables, once in a while, is a good salivary stimulant.

Food combinations: For best results one should abstain
                              from all beef and pork products. Do
not make a habit of eating even chicken, lamb, or fish every

[1]tbsp. = tablespoon.

day. Once a week or better, once a month is enough, if your system demands flesh foods at all. Nuts, cottage cheese, eggs, milk, cream, and bananas are very good meat and fish substitutes. If you eat chicken, lamb, or fish,[1] have a vegetable salad with them.

Fruit should be eaten with bread or some other starchy food, but without sugar; you may add a little honey if you wish. Eat only nature's candies (unsulphured figs, prunes or raisins).

Do not eat too much white sugar. The ingestion of excessive quantities of sweets causes intestinal fermentation.

Remember, foods prepared from white flour, such as white bread, white-flour gravy, etc., also polished rice and too many greasy fried foods, are injurious to your health.

Try to include in your daily diet as much raw food as possible. Cooked vegetables should be eaten with the juice in which they were boiled.

Catarrh of the alimentary canal often results from overeating at night, also from eating excessively of candy or other foodstuffs which have an irritating effect on the mucous membranes of the stomach, duodenum, etc.

Fast regularly, using your best judgment as to proper diet, in accordance with the instructions given above. Eat less, and follow dietary rules when you eat. Make sunshine, oxygen, and energy a part of your regular daily diet.

---

[1]Chicken, lamb, or fish should be thoroughly baked, stewed, or broiled, and eggs should be hard boiled before eating, in order to destroy any harmful bacteria which they may contain.

The daily diet: Your daily food intake should be chosen from the following list of foods which contain all the elements needed for the proper maintenance of the body:

½ apple
¼ grapefruit
1 lemon
1 lime
1 orange
1 glass orange juice with tbsp. finely ground nuts
1 small piece fresh pineapple
6 figs, dates, or prunes[1]
1 handful raisins[1]
1 tsp. honey
1 baked, or half-boiled or steamed vegetable with its juice
1 raw carrot, including part of green top
6 leaves raw spinach
¼ heart lettuce
1 tsp. olive oil
1 glass milk
⅛ glass cream
1 tbsp. cottage cheese
1 tbsp. clabber[2]

Eat at least some of the above foods every day, distributing them over your three meals. For instance, you may take the milk at breakfast, bread and egg and vegetable salad at noon, and the ground nuts and fruits at night.

Individual food habits may be taken into consideration, but if they are bad gradually change them. At any rate, add *some* of the foods in the above list to what you are used to eating. Omit those foods mentioned above which do not agree with you, eating only very lightly when you feel the

[1]These fruits are wholesome only when they are unsulphured. Ascertain that they are unsulphured before you buy them.
[2]Milk which has been allowed to stand in a warm place, preferably in an earthen vessel, for a day or longer, until it has soured or curdled.

7

need of nourishment, and gradually accustoming yourself to a more wholesome diet.

You may increase or decrease the quantities given above, in accordance with your individual needs. It is, of course, obvious that the person doing strenuous muscular work requires more food than the sedentary worker.

Whenever one is hungry one may take a large tablespoon-ful of thoroughly ground nuts in half a glass of water or in a glass of orange juice. When thirsty, drink a glass of orange juice or water (preferably distilled or boiled). However, nature's distilled water—undiluted fruit juice—is best. Do not drink too much ice water with meals. Ice water should be taken sparingly at any time, but especially during and after meals as it lowers the temperature of the stomach, thus retarding digestion. *Never drink ice water when you are overheated.*

THE MAGNETIC DIET

What distilled water is to a wet battery, food is to the body battery. The life energy in the body battery is derived from Cosmic Energy through the medulla, and from food. The life energy in the body breaks up the foods and converts them into energy also. It is the intricate task of the life force to distil more life force from the nourishment taken into the body. Therefore, one's dietary should be confined to foods which are easily converted into energy, or which are pro-ductive of fresh energy. Oxygen and sunshine should have a very important place in people's lives, because of their direct energy·producing quality. The more you depend on the will and on Cosmic Energy to sustain you, the less your food requirements; the more you depend on food, the weaker your will and the less your recourse to Cosmic Energy.

The magnetic diet consists of such food substitutes as rays and oxygen which can be easily assimilated and converted into energy by the latent life forces in the body. Magnetic foods give energy more quickly than solids and liquids which are less easily converted into life force.

When you are tired or hungry, take a sun bath, and you will find yourself recharged with ultraviolet rays, and re-vived; or inhale and exhale several times outdoors or near an open window, and your fatigue will be gone. A fasting per-son who inhales and exhales deeply twelve times, three times a day, recharges his body with electrons and free energy from air and ether. Contact of food and oxygen with the inner bodily system is necessary if the life force is to convert the food and oxygen into energy. The life force can assimilate oxygen more quickly than it can assimilate solids or liquids.

Practice the following exercise three times a day: Ex-hale slowly, counting from 1 to 6. Now, while the lungs are empty, mentally count from 1 to 6. Inhale slowly, count-ing from 1 to 6. Then hold the breath, counting from 1 to 6.[1] Repeat eleven times.

Just as electricity passes through a rod made of a con-ductive substance, and electrifies it, so the body battery be-comes fully charged with life force derived from oxygen.

[1]Never hold breath longer than it takes to count slowly from 1 to 6 or, at most, from 1 to 12.

People who perform breathing exercises always have shining, magnetic eyes.

One hour's sun bath is also a part of the magnetic diet.

The ultraviolet rays which one absorbs in one whole day on a bathing beach exert a beneficial vitalizing effect on the body, which lasts about three months. Sores and wounds can be cured by exposing them one-half hour daily to the sunlight.

Treatment with artificially produced ultraviolet and infra-red rays also supplies the body with magnetic nourishment. Much benefit may be derived from it if it is taken under the guidance of a specialist.

Ordinary window glass prevents the sun's ultraviolet rays from penetrating into a room.

Living in a sun room enclosed by yellow quartz glass, through which the ultraviolet sun rays penetrate, would supply the human body with magnetic spiritual nutriment and make it in turn spiritually magnetic. A man living in a room enclosed by red quartz glass would find brute force developing within himself.

Each one of the many billions of cells within the human body is a tiny mouth taking nourishment. The life force, identified with the body, creates within us a desire to derive energy from the circulation and from meat and other foods taken into the stomach. The life force must be trained to draw energy from subtler sources. The body's energy requirements can be supplied partly by sunshine and oxygen, which are absorbed by the pores. For this reason, the surface of the skin must be kept scrupulously clean at all times.

Exercising with will and concentration produces excellent results because it creates energy *directly,* by will development. This energy is quickly absorbed by the muscles, blood, bones, and sinews, for cellular rejuvenation. Therefore, the highest degree of energy accompanied by the least tissue destruction is derived from the Yogoda will exercises (Lessons 1 to 3).

Occasionally charging the body with electricity by holding on to two electrodes of a battery is a good method for supplying the body with free energy. (The electric current should be very weak.) Bathing in sunlight-heated or ultra-violet-ray-saturated water is very beneficial.

Rubbing the whole stripped body vigorously and rapidly with the palms before taking a bath generates life force and is also very beneficial.

If a weak man wrestles or lives in the same room with a strong, vital individual, he absorbs some of the latter's vital and mental magnetism. For this reason young and old people should mingle and thus exchange magnetism. Different people have different kinds of vitality. Always try to discover new methods for getting direct energy qualities from different individuals.

As a rule, the word "food" is used only in connection with material nourishment, but there are other kinds of food: mental energy, or concentration, and Divine Wisdom. The first (material food) recharges the body battery; the second (concentration), the mind battery; the third (Divine Wisdom), the soul battery.

11

Not only are proper material foods in the right combinations necessary for the sustenance of the body, but they exert a decided influence on the brain. The spiritual brain, the active brain, and the material brain are all affected by food, and can form different combinations: (1) spiritual-active brain, (2) intellectual-active brain, and (3) material-active brain.

All food that is eaten produces a sensation on the palate as well as certain chemical effects in body and brain. Food sensations determine a specific mentality. Foods such as dried meat produce gross material reactions which develop the material brain and animal mind. Likewise, the eating of active, vital foods, such as onions, garlic, fresh (not dried) meat, etc., produces an active brain. Eating raw fruits and vegetables produces spiritual qualities in the consumer and develops a spiritual mind and brain.

The quality of the food's taste and color is all reported to the brain through the nerves of taste and sight, and is experienced as specific pleasant or unpleasant sensations. These sensations are elaborated into perceptions and conceptions. Repeated conceptions about foods form definite mental habits and manifest themselves as material, active, or spiritual qualities.

While we know that material foods supply the body with energy, we must also remember that good thoughts are nourishing food for the mind, and thoughts of any other nature are poisonous to the health of body and mind.

Have you ever analyzed your magnetic mental diet? It consists usually of the thoughts which you are thinking as well

12

as the thoughts you are receiving from the close thought contact with your friends. Peaceful thoughts and peaceful friends always produce healthy, magnetic minds. It is easy to tell whether a person feeds on a quarrelsome or a peaceful environment. Inner disquietude and worries, due to the wrong sort of friends or unappreciative immediate relatives, produce an unwholesome, gloomy mind.

Ridding the mind *of worry poisons.* If you are suffering from mental ill health, go on a mental diet. A health-giving mental fast will clear the mind and rid it of the accumulated mental poisons resulting from a careless, faulty mental diet.

First of all, learn to remove the causes of your worries without permitting them to worry you. Do not feed your mind with daily created mental poisons of fresh worries.

Worries are often the result of attempting to do too many things hurriedly. Do not "bolt" your mental duties, but thoroughly masticate them, one at a time, with the teeth of attention and saturate them with the saliva of good judgment. Thus will you avoid worry indigestion.

Worry fasts. Then you must go on *worry fasts.* Three times a day shake off all worries. At seven o'clock in the morning say to yourself, "All my worries of the night are cast out, and from 7 to 8 A. M. I refuse to worry, no matter how troublesome are the duties ahead of me. I am going on a *worry fast.*"

13

From 12 to 1 P. M., say, "I am cheerful, I will not worry."

In the evening, between six and nine o'clock, while in the company of your husband or wife or "hard-to-get-along-with" relatives or friends, mentally make a strong resolution and say, "Within these three hours I will not worry, I refuse to get vexed, even if I am nagged. No matter how tempting it is to indulge in a *worry feast,* I will resist the temptation. I have been very sick of worries—my heart of peace has been diseased. I have had several worry heart attacks. I must not paralyze and kill my peace-heart by shocks of worries. I am on a *worry fast.* I cannot afford to worry."

After you succeed in carrying out *worry fasts* during certain hours of the day, try doing it for a week or two weeks at a time, and then try to prevent the accumulation of worry poisons in your system, entirely.

Whenever you find yourself indulging in a *worry feast,* go on a partial or complete *worry fast* for a day or a week.

Whenever you make up your mind not to worry, *i.e.,* to go on a *worry fast, stick to your resolution.* You can stop worrying entirely. You can calmly solve your most difficult problems, putting forth your greatest effort, and at the same time absolutely refuse to worry. Tell your mind, "I can do only my best; no more. I am satisfied and happy that I *am* doing my best to solve my problem; there is absolutely no reason why I should worry myself to death."

When you are on a *worry fast,* you need not be in a negative mental state. Drink copiously of the fresh waters of peace flowing from the spring of every circumstance, vital-

14

ized by your determination to be cheerful. If you have made up your mind to be cheerful, nothing can make you unhappy. If you do not choose to destroy your own peace of mind by accepting the suggestion of unhappy circumstances, none can make you dejected. You are concerned only with the untiring performance of right *actions* for right results; but your whole attention must be on the actions, and not on their results. Leave the latter to God, saying, "I have done my best under the circumstances. Therefore, I am happy."

Joy as a cure for worry. The negative method for overcoming worry poisoning is *worry fasting*. There are also positive methods. One infected with the germs of worry must go on a strict mental diet. He must feast frugally, but regularly, on the society of joyful minds. Every day he must associate—if only for a little while—with "joy-infected" minds. There are some people the song of whose laughter nothing can still. Seek them out and feast with them on this most vitalizing food of joy. Continue the laughter diet for a month or two. Feast on laughter in the company of really joyful people. Digest it thoroughly by whole-heartedly masticating laughter with the teeth of your attention. Steadfastly continue your laughter diet once you have begun it, and at the end of a month or two you will see the change—your mind will be filled with sunshine. Remember, specific habits can be cultivated only by specific habit-forming actions.

15

The courage diet: Having benefited by the *worry fast,*
                        try the *fear fast* next, going on a courage
diet for certain hours, days, or weeks. You must act spiritually in order to be spiritual.

The wisdom diet: In order to destroy ignorance, go on
                       a *wisdom diet.* Drink the tonic of wis-
dom from the lips of intuition. You can learn from intuition
when you meet it in the chamber of deep meditation. Read
good books of a devotional and spiritual nature, taking from
them what you need.

Consult a spiritual specialist. If your disease of ignorance
is chronic, be guided entirely by him. That patient cannot
be cured who depends only on his own judgment which may
be affected by his state of mental ill health.

Go on ignorance-elimination fasts. Refuse to be enslaved
by ignorant habits and thoughtless actions. Take up intensive spiritual study and intensive spiritual dieting, and
refuse to suffer any longer from the infection of ignorance.

Overcoming mental   Mental stagnation is "mental T. B."
stagnation.   Come out of your closed chamber of
                      narrowness. Drink in the fresh air of
others' vital thoughts and views. Drink vitality; receive
mental nourishment from materially and spiritually progressive minds. Feast unstintingly on the creative thinking
within yourself and others. Take long mental walks on the
paths of self-confidence. Exercise with the instruments of
judgment, introspection, and initiative. Exhale poisonous

16

thoughts of discouragement, discontentment, hopelessness, etc. Inhale the fresh oxygen of success, and know that you are progressing with God's help. This will recharge your soul battery. By consciously experiencing God's Bliss through meditation, you can consciously destroy mental stagnation and acquire progressive spiritual health and wisdom.

Acquiring physical, mental, and spiritual perfection. Thus, day by day, eating spiritual magnetism-producing foods and absorbing vitality-producing sunshine, you will physically reflect God's everlasting youth. Eliminating all mental poisons and partaking of the divine nourishment of determination, courage, continuous, unfailing mental effort and concentration, you will learn to overcome the most difficult problems with ease. Eliminating ignorance by constant meditation on God, and following the precepts of Yogoda and your spiritual teacher, you will attain perfect spiritual health. Once you acquire this spiritual health, you will give your life to and for others, to show them also the way to supreme, intoxicating spiritual health.

Once you learn to eat right foods, think right thoughts, being filled with wisdom and joy, your body, mind, and soul will be spiritualized and perceived as dynamos of magnetic energy. Your body and mind, purified by this energy, will take on the beauty of the Spirit. Once you realize yourself as a soul, you will know you are of the Spirit, resting every-

17

where equally in joy, in all space, in all things, as one with all things.

A body, mind, and soul magnet, recharged with good food, rays, power, wisdom, and Bliss, draws unto itself all material and spiritual souls, spiritually deeply magnetic, like itself. A spiritual magnet is charged with the life of God, and whomsoever it touches it makes God of him.

SUMMARY

Those who think that life depends only on breakfast, lunch and dinner—on solids and liquids—are gross-minded. We can derive energy either from material foods or from the Cosmic Source.

The man of the future will draw nourishment from the ether and from the ocean of invisible Cosmic Energy in which he moves and has his being.

It is the aim of this lesson:

(1) To direct the student's attention to the advisability of drawing his energy requirements, so far as possible, from air and sunlight. The nourishment derived from these two sources can be most easily converted into energy within the body.

(2) To show the student the necessity of choosing only those material foods which emit and lodge spiritual vibrations in man's mind and brain.

Material foods impress the mind with certain good or bad qualities, and people's thoughts, actions, and health generally are determined by the foods they eat.

18

Super-Advanced Course No. 1

·•·❖·•·

Lesson No. 6

·•·❖·•·

INSTALLING HABITS
OF SUCCESS, HEALTH, AND WISDOM
IN THE MIND AT WILL

By

SWAMI YOGANANDA

·•·❖·•·

This sacred lesson is meant only for the devoted Yogoda
student who would, untiringly and unceasingly,
seek God until he finds Him

·•·❖·•·

Published By
YOGODA SAT-SANGA SOCIETY
3880 San Rafael Avenue
Mount Washington
Los Angeles, Calif.

Cosmic Law   In search for success one must con-
and "needs."   centrate on "needs" and not on "wants."

It is well that man does not get every-
thing he wants, and that the Cosmic Law does not grant the
wishes which would result in harm. A child may ask his
father to catch him a beautiful poisonous snake, but the
father does not fulfill such a dangerous wish. The Divine
Law also denies the gratification of harmful, though momentarily pleasurable, desires. Of course, man, as the free-born
child of God, can, and often does, persist in his longing for
something quite delightful in the beginning but harmful in
the end.

The greater the need, the greater the likelihood that it will
be filled.

Before you can get that which you want, you must develop the power to get *at will* that which you need.

How to find true   What are your real needs? Shelter;
happiness.   food for body, mind, and soul; pros-
                       perity; health; the power of concentra-
tion; a good memory; an understanding heart; friends; wisdom, and Bliss, are some human needs. Plain living, high
thinking, cultivating real happiness within oneself in order
to make others spiritually happy, are also real needs. True
happiness is lasting, because it is spiritual in nature, whereas
the "happiness" based on sense pleasure soon turns to sorrow. Making the senses serve the needs of body and mind
leads to true happiness; indulging the senses brings nothing
but misery. A desire for a pleasurable sense object is often
mistaken for a natural "need" instead of an artificially cre-

1

ated "want." "Wants" must not be multiplied; instead, the whole of concentration must be directed toward the filling of real "needs" or the securing of actual necessities.

As a rule, the attention is absorbed by loosely floating, unnecessary "wants" and constantly increasing desires. All desires for the gratification of needless "wants" must be stamped out.

Focusing the attention on one "need" at a time is the first step in the right direction. Determine your greatest "need," involving all the factors of life and true happiness; then devote all your attention and energy to attaining your objective by the quickest method.

Human lives are governed not by weak resolutions, but by habits. When people are used to good health, prosperity, a high standard of living, writing, lecturing, etc., all these seem to come easily. Likewise, poverty and failure come to those who are used to them.

Actions of habit, good or bad, are performed easily and naturally, bringing about good or bad results. *Success and failure are habits.* Therefore, if you are used to poverty or sickness, you must learn how to get used to health and prosperity instead. If failure, sickness, and ignorance are your constant companions, *nothing but lack of will* prevents you from enlisting the aid of success, health, and knowledge to drive and keep them away, definitely and permanently.

The soul's heritage.   Success, health, and wisdom are the natural attributes and habits of the soul. Identification with constantly manifested *weak* habits and thoughts, and lack of concentration, per-

2

severance and courage are responsible for the misery which people suffer due to poverty, ill health, and so forth.

You are paralyzing your faculty for success by thoughts of fear. Success and perfection of mind and body are man's inherent qualities, *because he is made in God's image. In order to be able to claim his birthright, however, he must first rid himself of the delusion of his own limitations.*

God owns everything. Therefore, know at all times that *you, as God's child, own everything that belongs to the Father.* The whole mental attitude of an individual must be that of a son of God who is fully satisfied and contented, because he knows he has access to all his Father's possessions. Your native endowment is perfection and prosperity, but you choose to be imperfect and poor. *This sense of possessing everything must be a mental habit with each individual.*

Of what use are habits to us? Habit formation is a device given us for the easy performance of certain actions. Habits are mental mechanisms which enable us to act automatically, leaving our consciousness free for other duties. A habit is formed by several attentive repetitions of an action.

Time required for habit formation can be shortened. A special mental note should be made here about slow or rapid habit formation. Some people require much time to form mental habits of health, prosperity, and the acquirement of wisdom. Actually, the time

3

needed for this purpose can be shortened. Slow or rapid habit formation depends on the general state of health; on the condition of the nervous system, including that of the brain cells; on habit-forming methods, mental imagery, will, etc. When a wholesome mental attitude is a strong habit—strong enough to be unshakable—no matter how many times you become ill, you will recover. Most people are "half-hearted" in their thoughts and actions; hence they do not succeed.

A mental habit, in order to materialize, must be strong and persistent.

For instance, the health or prosperity habit must be cultivated by health or prosperity thoughts until results are apparent. An unfailingly wholesome, courageous mental attitude is absolutely necessary to the attainment of one's "needs" and "wants." Failure to prosper and be healthy is due unquestionably to weak mental habits of health and prosperity.

Dislodge negative thoughts. In affirming, "I am healthy," or "I am wise," the positive affirmation must be so strong that it crowds out completely any subconscious, discouraging, negative enemy thoughts which may be whispering to you, "you fool, you will never succeed. You are a failure; wisdom is impossible for you." You must *know* that whatever you wish strongly, you can materialize in short order.

4

Disregard the In practicing affirmations, the spirit-
time element ual aspirant must be unfailingly patient.
while affirming. *Believe you are inherently healthy when*
you want good health; believe you are
inherently prosperous when you want prosperity; believe
you are inherently wise when you want wisdom—then
health, prosperity, and wisdom will manifest themselves in
you.

Change the trend of your thoughts; cast out all negative
mental habits, substituting in their place wholesome, courageous thought habits, and *applying them in daily life, with*
unshakable confidence.

Remember that while an inattentive, scatter-brained idiot
requires a long time for the formation of even a simple habit,
an intelligent, purposeful individual can easily form or substitute a good mental habit for a bad one, in a trice, by the
mere wish. Therefore, if you have a habit—mental, physical, or spiritual—that impedes your progress, *rid yourself of*
it now; do not put it off.

Exercises: (A) If you are afflicted with a
chronic case of indifference, make up
your mind at once to "snap out of it." Be gay; think of
something amusing until you find yourself bubbling over
with laughter. Exercise self-control; learn to substitute, at
will, joy for sorrow; love for hate; courage for fear; open-
mindedness for prejudice.

(B)   Know that anything others can do, you can do also.[1]

(C)   If you have an inferiority complex, remember that success, health, and wisdom are your rightful heritage. Your difficulty is due to weakness which may have had its inception in one or more factors. It can be overcome by determination, courage, common sense, and faith in God and in yourself.

Therefore, if you are firmly convinced you are a failure, change your mental attitude at once; be unshakable in your conviction that you have all the potentialities of great success. At times you may find it helpful to recall your mental reactions on occasions when you were successful in some undertaking.

Practice the fourth Yogoda lesson faithfully and regularly and consult your spiritual teacher.

---

[1]Once I was having dinner with friends. Everything went well until the Roquefort cheese was served. In India we eat only freshly made cheese, so I viewed the little green specks of mold in the cheese with great suspicion. My soul rebelled against it, and my brain cells warned me to have nothing to do with it. But as I looked at my American friends eating the cheese, I mustered courage and took a lump of it into my mouth. No sooner had it landed there than all the aristocratic delicacies which had preceded it rebelled. There was great clamor and commotion within me, and they served notice on me that if "Mr. Roquefort" joined them they would all leave in a body. And I dared not open my mouth, but just nodded in answer to my host's question whether I liked the cheese! Then, as I looked intently at the faces of my friends eating Roquefort cheese pleasantly, I suddenly made up my mind. Concentrating deeply, I told my brain cells, "I am your 'boss': you are my servants. You shall obey me—this foolishness must stop." The next minute I was enjoying "Mr. Roquefort's" company pleasantly, and now he always receives a warm welcome when he enters my "hall of digestion."

6

You may find it necessary also to change your mental and physical environment in order to install the proper habits of thought.

After you begin to experience success, act with wisdom and perseverance, no matter what happens, until you demonstrate that you have succeeded just as you believed you would if you tried.

SUMMARY

It does not take long to develop good mental habits. In fact, by exercising strong will, mental habits of health or success or wisdom may be formed at once. By concentrating with perseverance, courage, and faith in God and oneself on legitimate necessities, one can materialize them at will.

Super-Advanced Course No. 1

—+—

Lesson No. 7

—+—

MAGNETISM

By

SWAMI YOGANANDA

—+—

This sacred lesson is meant only for the devoted Yogoda
student who would, untiringly and unceasingly,
seek God until he finds Him

—+—

Published By
YOGODA SAT-SANGA SOCIETY
3830 San Rafael Avenue
Mount Washington
Los Angeles, Calif.

What is   The definitions of magnetism are, on
magnetism?   the whole, quite similar. The following
                       are typical: Magnetism is (1) that prop-
erty possessed by various bodies . . . of attracting or repelling each other; (2) the force to which this attraction is
due; (3) the science that treats of the laws of this force;
(4) personal attraction or charm . . .[1] There is also what
is known as animal magnetism, hypnotism, and so forth.

Now let us see what can be learned about magnetism by
an intuitional, metaphysical study, which differs from the
investigations of physical science in its ability to scale dimen-
sional boundaries.

Originally there was nothing but Undifferentiated Spirit.
In order to make possible the creation of dualities and multi-
farious objects, Spirit had to project; that is, fling forth
vibratory force. This repulsed force became Cosmic Energy,
out of which the universe and all that is in it materialized.

The origin   After the universal creative force
of evil.   "fell from heaven"—after it was cast
                       out of the bosom of the Cosmic Spirit
and became independent—it began creating delusive, finite
dualities contrary to the pattern of the Spirit. In the Spirit
was perfection when It was divided into the many. The
part could not manifest the quality of the whole. *This conscious, independent force is "Satan," or the satanic creator
of all evil and misery-producing finite objects.*

[1] The Winston Simplified Dictionary, Advanced edition, page 589.

1

Why we are bound to matter. Satan wants everything to *reincarnate* and remain in its finite state through the laws of material attachment, instinct, desire, and so forth. If this force were not conscious, human beings—in fact, all creation—after a certain interval would be able to cast off Satan's bonds and return to Spirit. Because Satan deludes all creatures with the consciousness of finiteness and unspiritual duality, they must go through the process of evolution. Thus, souls must reincarnate through the law of cause and effect, and the power of desire born of contact with finite matter.

What is spiritual magnetism? The Spirit, through Its force of universal attraction, is gradually absorbing all objects created out of It by the misguided force of satanic delusion. In other words, living beings and souls have allowed themselves to be lured away from God and become attached to matter through the influence of the creative force projected by God, who is calling His truant children back to Himself.

The tug-of-war of divine and evil forces in man. Satan is opposing Spirit's emancipating magnetism which expresses itself in all of creation as an urge toward perfection. Each individual feels within himself the tug-of-war between God's attracting, divine magnetism and Satan's outwardly repelling magnetism. Satanic magnetism keeps objects attracted to matter. Through man's discriminating and intuitive faculties he feels and re-

2

sponds to the call of Spirit, while through his senses and mind he is drawn to matter.

KINDS OF MAGNETISM

Electronic magnetism. Electrons and protons are held together to a nucleus by the power of universal magnetism. This is termed electronic magnetism. Because the Spirit is in everything and possesses this drawing power, all things created out of It also have the individuality of the Spirit and Its drawing magnetic power which pervades every heart, permeates all things.

Solar magnetism. The sun's power of attraction, which causes the planets to revolve around it, is called solar magnetism.

Atomic and molecular magnetism. All atoms and molecules have a nucleus which holds their tiny particles together. The cohesive power in atom and molecule is called atomic magnetism and molecular magnetism, respectively.

Chemical magnetism. The power that holds together the constituents of, say, H_2SO_4, or sulphuric acid, is called chemical magnetism.

Material magnetism. The power that holds together the rocks and like natural objects is called material magnetism.

3

Plant magnetism.	The power within plants, which draws nourishment out of air and sod and keeps plants from disintegrating is termed plant magnetism.
Animal magnetism.	Animal organisms are held together by animal magnetism. Animals also have within themselves the power by

which they attract other animals. The snake, for example, charms and draws little animals to itself by its animal magnetic power.

Magnetism in man.	Man, being a rational, esthetic, spiritual animal, possesses intellectual, moral, esthetic and spiritual as well as animal magnetism.

The right kind of magnetic power has expanding, uplifting and spiritual qualities. Some people are so magnetic that they inspire us and expand our consciousness. This is the sort of magnetic power that we all want, not the stupefying kind of hypnotic or animal magnetism.

Hypnotism vs. spiritual magnetism.	Hypnotism is a spiritual crime, as the hypnotist robs his subject of free will, judgment and consciousness. An individual under the influence of hypnotism

is unconscious of his surroundings and aware only of the suggestions of the hypnotist. The conscious mind of the hypnotized person is inert. A person upon whom hypnotism is practiced repeatedly for any great length of time be-

4

comes weak-willed and loses all natural forcefulness, being guided by enslaving suggestions.

Never permit yourself to be influenced by anyone's animal magnetism or semi-hypnotic power, which differs but slightly from hypnotism. When an individual exercises his animal magnetism over another, his subject is blinded and unable to perceive clearly the danger to which he is exposed. A person so influenced may *seem* to be a free agent, but in reality he is guided entirely by another's instincts and habits.

HOW TO DEVELOP MORAL, ESTHETIC, BUSINESS, SPIRITUAL, AND DIVINE MAGNETISM

As you know, a magnet has a positive and a negative pole through which it draws toward itself pieces of iron or steel within a certain range. When a magnet is rubbed against a piece of non-magnetic iron or steel, the latter also becomes magnetic. People, too, can become magnetized through close association with magnetic personalities to whom they give their deep, loving, respectful attention. They should, however, first decide what kind of magnetism they want and then choose the particular persons who possess it.

Exchanging magnetism in shaking hands. For instance, if you are a failure and you want success, associate and shake hands as much as possible with those who have attained success in their business, art, or profession. (Of course, it is not always easy to make such contacts, but "where there's a will, there's a way.")

5

In shaking hands, two magnets are formed: the upper—spiritual—magnet with the two heads, and the lower—physical—magnet with the two pairs of feet as poles. The junction of the hands in the handshake forms the common neutral point as well as the curve for the upper and lower magnets.

Let us see what happens when a spiritual man, who is a failure, and a prosperous business man, who is spiritually weak, attentively shake hands. Through the two pairs of feet, forming the two poles of one magnet, they exchange physical qualities; and through the two heads, forming the two poles of another magnet, they exchange mental qualities. If such men come in close mental contact, besides shaking hands frequently and attentively, the business man becomes more spiritual and the spiritual man becomes more prosperous, by virtue of the upper magnet. They exchange their bad qualities also, through the power of the lower magnet formed by the feet. Both the spiritual man and the business man may be affected in their vocational qualities.

We will now take a different case, that of a reformer of weak character who endeavors to influence a stubborn, confirmed evildoer, by close association and oft-repeated handshaking. It is quite likely that the reformer will become a positive pole, drawing evil qualities, and the evildoer will become a negative pole, passively drawing good qualities in a very limited way. In this case, the reformer would be the one to be changed. Therefore, unless one has grown very strong spiritually, he should not attempt to reform the very wicked.

From the foregoing, it becomes evident that *indiscriminate handshaking may prove detrimental.* It is harmful to associate constantly with undesirable individuals with whom frequent handshaking is unavoidable, though an occasional handshake is not of much consequence and may be necessary for courtesy's sake.

Young people of opposite sex, living on the material plane, often exchange animal magnetism, blind one another by emotions and passions, and draw unto themselves all kinds of destructive, evil mentalities.

The range of influence of material magnetism is very low except in unusual cases. Successful business men can but rarely influence failures from a distance.

For the purpose of exchanging moral, mental, esthetic, or spiritual magnetism, personal contact is not always necessary. When one visualizes a spiritual man and deeply meditates on his mentality and character, one can attract and imitate his spiritual magnetism.

Developing spiritual magnetism by self-effort. One who continually lives, thinks and dreams of spirituality and friendship, contacts the Spirit's own magnetism and feels Its ennobling influence. One who meditates on Om and God day and night and intuitively perceives all-attracting Divine Magnetism, develops spiritual magnetism of limitless range and power and can draw unto himself whatever he wants, uplifting people either by personal contact or from afar, through his powerfully directed concentration. By this power, one is able to draw unto himself his true friends from previous incarnations; he can command the elements to do his bidding; he can draw all creative, luminous forces, and can invite angels, saints and savants who have passed on, to come to him and dance in his joy. Such a person can attract to himself the rays of all knowledge so that they will sparkle and scintillate around his being.

DIVINE LOVE SORROWS

I have been roaming,
Forsaken by Thee—
Who have seen me groping,
Hardly ever answering.
I shall be roaming, roaming,
    Bursting all boundaries of heart,
Evermore moving toward Thee,
    To Thy vast unthrobbing heart.

Come, Thou, to me, O Lord!
    Oh, come at last to me.
Centuries and centuries
    I have waited now for Thee.
Through endless incarnations
    I called out for Thy name,
Searching by the streamlets
    Of all my silvery dreams.

I knew that Thou must come at last
To steal the flowers of my heart.
In sorrow thrills I piped my love;
I sadly sang my song to Thee.
And yet I knew my love must reach Thee,
Though many lives I had to wait;
On mountain crags of high devotion,
I sadly sang my song, my song, my song.

———

THOU AND I, MY LORD

So be Thou, my Lord,
Thou and I, never apart;
Wave of the sea,
Dissolve in the sea.
I am the bubble,
Make me the sea!

9

FORMULAS FOR THE DEVELOPMENT OF MAGNETISM BETWEEN INDIVIDUALS OF DIFFERENT MATERIAL, MENTAL AND SPIRITUAL QUALITIES

CONTACTING ELEMENTS	PREDOMINATING TRAITS OF THE TWO INDIVIDUALS	Predominant Magnetism Resulting from Frequent Close Contact
GOOD AND EVIL	Strongly positive evil + passively negative good. Weakly negative evil + strongly positive good.	Positive evil. Positive good.
IRASCIBILITY AND TRANQUILLITY	Marked irascibility + negative mildness. Negative calmness + slight irascibility.	Marked irascibility. Tranquillity.
FAILURE AND SUCCESS	Strongly positive failure + less positive failure. Strongly positive success + less positive success. Strongly positive failure + strongly positive success.	Confirmed failure. Confirmed success. Either failure or success.
BUSINESS AND SPIRITUAL WORK	Strongly positive spirituality + strongly positive business success.	Strongly positive business success and spirituality.
INTELLIGENCE AND STUPIDITY	Strongly positive intelligence + marked stupidity. Strongly positive intelligence + negative intelligence.	Either intelligence or stupidity. Str. positive intelligence.

Super-Advanced Course No. 1

·•·✠·•·

Lesson No. 8

·•·✠·•·

OBLITERATING THE MALIGNANT SEEDS
OF FAILURE AND ILL HEALTH
FROM THE SUBCONSCIOUS MIND

By

SWAMI YOGANANDA

·•·✠·•·

This sacred lesson is meant only for the devoted Yogoda
student who would, untiringly and unceasingly,
seek God until he finds Him

·•·✠·•·

Published By
YOGODA SAT-SANGA SOCIETY
3880 San Rafael Avenue
Mount Washington
Los Angeles, Calif.

The ultimate purpose of man's presence in the world of matter is *the attainment of spiritual perfection.* Once his development reaches that state, he can cast off the shackles of perishable matter and join God in the realm of Eternal Bliss.

Are ill health and failure accidents? It is man's reaction to his various experiences—the manner in which he passes his tests in the school of life—which indicates how far he has advanced toward perfection. Let us bear in mind that *the consequences produced by his reactions to every-day experiences not only affect his progress toward ultimate eternal freedom, but they also determine his health or sickness, his success or failure for many incarnations.* Like some physical diseases which send their roots deep into his body, the evil effects of man's actions, unless destroyed, become a part of his conscious, subconscious and super-consciousness, and are felt not alone in one lifetime, but in many lives.

What causes good or ill fortune? The failures and successes of every-day life become rooted in the mind. Unless they come to fruition or are worked out by wisdom, they bear seeds which the soul must carry over into another incarnation as tendencies and traits. These stubborn ghosts of the past are hiding in the recesses of your mind, emerging suddenly to help and inspire or hinder and discourage, according to the circumstances confronting you. It is for this reason

1

that so many people fail in their undertakings, in spite of their conscious efforts.

From the viewpoint of material science, personal traits and tendencies are due merely to the accident of one's birth into a family of which such traits and tendencies are characteristic. This is very limiting and unsatisfactory. Why should *we* be made to suffer for the sins of our forefathers? On the other hand, why should we be blindly endowed with health, wealth, or genius, *without effort on our part?* To an unseeing materialist, disease, health, wealth or genius may appear to be just the results of a physical law of cause and effect, or hereditary weakness or contagion or good fortune. When a physician discovers a tubercular infection in a patient whose history shows that several members of preceding generations of his immediate family died from this disease, he is convinced that the patient has inherited a natural tendency for tuberculosis. The metaphysician, who attempts to trace the deeper causes of diseases and apparently unjust suffering, finds that the so-called hereditary diseases and predispositions do not come to anyone accidentally. Rather, a disembodied soul carrying a tubercular tendency from a previous existence is born into a family in in which there is tubercular infection.

How to escape the results of wrong actions.   Of course, tuberculosis can also be contracted by a healthy person who disregards all physical and hygienic laws. However well, good or prosperous one may be, he cannot be sure of his behavior or future unless

2

he has destroyed all seeds of disease-and-failure-producing actions of the past. This is by no means easy, but it can be done. (We shall see presently what means must be taken toward that end.)

The one certain method for escaping the results of a specific action is to destroy it in this life; otherwise, it will be carried over into the next incarnation. The most successful financier, the healthiest of men, the most intolerant self-righteous moralist—all are liable to be humbled by the sudden manifestation of *failure tendencies, hidden germ notions of disease,* and *unsuspected weaknesses.*

It has been said that Henry Ford, during the war, nearly lost everything—his whole vast fortune. He had acquired great wealth because he had been prosperous in former lives, but his mind was also filled with fears of failure and the failures of past lives, so, during the war, while conditions at times were unfavorable to certain lines of business, his failure seeds sprouted and almost caused his financial ruin. If he had permitted himself to become truly discouraged he would have lost everything. By a superhuman effort of will, he fought off his brutal business competitors who were bent on destroying the organization he had built up during many years of hard work. His success consciousness of the past was reinforced by his initiative in this life, by his trained business judgment, his knack for choosing the right workers for his organization, his perseverance, and his daring.

To summarize it briefly, financial success, metaphysically speaking, depends on one's earning ability in past lives and one's initiative and painstaking and persevering quality of

3

will in this life. To raise false hopes on the one hand or discourage an ambitious person on the other, is wrong—the real metaphysician determines the exact influence of the prosperity seeds of past actions and the quality and degree of prosperity will-effort during this life.

How our actions If the success tendency from a past
of the past and life and the efforts to succeed in this
present affect life are weak, then the chances of finan-
our lives. cial success in this incarnation are mea-
gre; in fact, they are almost negligible. If a person's success tendency from a past life is strong, and present life is marked by inactivity and inertia, then he will either be born into a wealthy family or suddenly inherit a fortune. Some individuals who became indifferent to their wealth in the preceding incarnation may be reborn amidst poverty and struggle, only to acquire great wealth by a so-called "stroke of luck," or through a sudden inheritance, or through lucky small investments.

The individual who has a strong prosperity consciousness from a past life and makes a strenuous effort to earn money in this life succeeds in all his ventures; such a person seldom loses an investment and has unfailing business judgment. If one starts out with a poverty tendency from previous lives but makes an earnest effort to overcome it in this life, he finds that he has to struggle uphill in order to succeed. He may either become prosperous late in life or die struggling. But don't think that his efforts have been in vain, for his next incarnation will be dominated by the success *Karma* resulting from those struggles. Those who "give up" and accept failure as the decree of fate are foolish, for success or failure is the result of acquirement either of the present or of the past. If you did not acquire wealth before, or if you did acquire it and lost it, dying with the consciousness of your loss, you are reborn in poverty. *By putting up a struggle to overcome your handicap, you stimulate all the dormant success consciousness of past lives, until it becomes active and overshadows the influence of the predominating failure tendencies.*

The will is man's most effective weapon in the battle of life. A man cannot be an absolute failure unless he permits his cowardly fears of failure to exert their paralyzing influence over him until nothing can convince him that he can ever again succeed.

Friendly success tendencies are ready to help an individual, and inimical failure tendencies to crush him, depending in the first case on his unflinching efforts, and in the second on his attitude of resignation to "his fate." These are his invisible friends and also his unseen enemies. Let him rouse his will by repeated judicious efforts, and ultimately he is sure to awaken the success tendencies sleeping in the dark chamber of subconsciousness. The will is the weapon by means of which he can vanquish failure. He must, however, make constant use of it; then it will always be sharp and keen-edged and serve him faithfully. The power of a strong will, *guided by divine wisdom,* is unlimited. To its possessor nothing is impossible.

The complexities of life and man's weakness, which places him at the mercy of the conflicting tendencies within himself, keep him from being successful in all lives. No one is a financial success or failure in all lives, for success and failure are the results of "heredity" (i.e., seed tendencies from past lives) and environment—the latter, of course, being determined by the former, and the influence of both, by the strength or weakness of man's will. Man has erred much and carries within himself the seeds of those errors. We must not forget, however, that he also carries within the seeds of all fulfillment. Under favorable conditions these germinate, and their growth helps to choke the weeds of failure. Hence it becomes evident that real financial success in all lives, until emancipation is achieved, is not impossible to one who knows how to destroy the tendencies of failure by the power of super-concentration.

A Yogi may not have many material possessions, but by his ability to focus his mind he learns to create at will the financial success he needs. (Of course, the Yogi does not entertain selfish desires; his only wish is that "God's love reign in the shrine of his soul forever.") True Yogis pray, "Heavenly Father! May we kindle Thy love in the flaming heart-altars of others."

When Yogis desire financial success for the group of individuals in a spiritual organization or for a single individual, they put on the success and failure tendencies of the past lives of the person or persons involved, and have to struggle like other people to gain their objective. However, the Yogi's good will always quickens the success of others.

6

The only possibility of abolishing want lies in the willingness of successful people to aid failures by helping them overcome their past *Karma* and stimulating their discouraged initiative. Some satisfy their craving for wealth by impoverishing their fellowmen; others fail to share their prosperity. Their selfishness is responsible for much suffering in this world. It is deplorable that people who ride in Rolls Royces often utterly disregard the needs of thousands of mental and physical cripples who have never received the help that would enable them to help themselves.

A wealthy man who has acquired success by overcoming his failure tendencies, becoming lazy or ignoring the agonies and needs of others, may lose his wealth through poor investments or attract poverty to himself in the next life. Heedless rich people who disregard the sufferings of others are reborn with a craving for luxuries but lack the means to satisfy that craving.

The seeds of wrong actions can be burned and the growth of seeds of good actions stimulated by the faithful practice of meditation. A man striving for permanent success must meditate every morning and night, and when the superconscious peace-and-concentration rays break through the nocturnal blackness of restlessness, he must concentrate these rays on the brain and mind, scorching out the lurking seeds of past failures and stimulating the success tendencies.

During meditation the Yogi feels the power of concentration in the will centre, i.e., at the point between the eyebrows, and also experiences

7

a feeling of complete peace throughout his body. Whenever he wants to scour from the brain cells the seeds of past failure or sickness, he must turn that peace-and-concentration power on the whole brain. The entire peace feeling of the body as well as the power of concentration felt between the eyebrows must be transferred and felt in the entire brain. In this way the brain cells become impregnated with peace and power, and their chemical and psychological hereditary composition is modified.

The practice of Yogoda exercises, concentration and meditation, destroy the seeds of disease. For the purpose of burning seeds of lurking and chronic diseases, the body-battery recharging Yogoda exercises of Lesson 1, Exercises B, must be practiced with deep concentration and followed by Lessons 4 and 5. In practicing Lessons 4 and 5, the consciousness of health, energy, and power must be kept predominating. When this power is felt all over the body as an unquenchable flow of vitality, it must be concentrated on the brain and mind uninterruptedly for a long time. In this way the vital power will destroy all lurking disease tendencies from the past.

There are many types or degrees of health and disease. Let us examine a few of them and trace their past *Karmas*, diagnosing their prenatal and postnatal habits:

The "asbestos" type of health.

"Asbestos Clan." Some few people enjoy such perfect, glowing health that they may be said to belong to the water-and-fireproof "Asbestos Clan." This is due to the accumulated health

8

habits of many lives (including the last incarnation), and to obeying health laws and exercising regularly in this incarnation. As a rule this type of individual has been a Yogi in many lives and can destroy all seeds of ill health so long as he practices Yoga.[1] If he confines himself merely to obeying health laws, *i.e.,* if he exercises regularly, eats properly, etc., but fails to practice Yoga, he *may* retain his health, but stands a chance of losing it late in life. The one who faithfully and correctly practices Yoga concentration and meditation as taught in the fourth and fifth lessons thereby kills the seeds of his little health transgressions. The aspirant for the "asbestos" type of health should not be satisfied to depend merely on the health tendencies of the past and on physical exercise in this life, but should also burn the accumulating seeds of unhealthy actions of this life, no matter how insignificant they may seem.

The "born-   Some people are in good health nearly
healthy" type.   all the time, but when they are sick they
                      are violently sick. Health of this type
is due to accumulated health seed tendencies and to ordinary care and exercise in this life, but not to Yoga practices. Health gives way when that which has been accumulated is used up. At such time the little transgression seeds of life become active and troublesome.

The "medium-   Individuals of this type are healthy
health" type.   but weak. The exercise of will power
                      results in the health seed tendencies

[1]Yoga: Communion with God through the practice of scientific meditation.

9

which produce "medium health." Physical exercise will prove strengthening.

The "mechanical-health" type. The health of persons of this type is like the mechanism of a fine watch—excellent with proper care, but trouble-some at the slightest neglect. They are well only so long as they follow rules; as soon as they break them they suf-fer. So much dependence on law, instead of faith in God and self-reliance, makes people health-law bound. They are victims of the "law complex." Do not permit laws to enslave you; use them to serve you.

The "die-hard" type. Some continue to exist in spite of a hailstorm of disease. Their health and disease tendencies are evenly balanced; hence they alternate between health and illness. If you have great devotion and are obedient to God's laws, He is much more likely to respond than if you have great devo-tion but constantly break His hygienic, mental and spir-itual laws.

The "convales-cent" type. There are some whose constitutions are as delicate and fragile as that of a flower. They cannot stand the slight-est hardship. This is due to their burning the seeds of dis-ease late in the preceding incarnation. In other words, death occurred after the seeds of ill health were destroyed late in life. Such people are born frail, because the circum-

10

stances connected with their recovery are still fresh in their memories; yet *they are healthy.*

Why do great souls—those who have attained spiritual perfec-tion—suffer? Sometimes great teachers suffer ill health and poverty because of their ef-forts to free their fellowmen from the clutches of disease and want. They sac-rifice their bodies and possessions and devote their minds solely to the task of helping others escape the fruits of their past errors. Jesus sacrificed His life that He might help suffering, error-stricken humanity to spiritual freedom. The Buddha gave up wealth, position, family—in short, all earthly possessions —for the same purpose. Great souls do this of their own accord, for God does not compel them to make this sacrifice.

When all the seeds of evil tendencies have been de-stroyed, each microscopic brain cell will be filled with wisdom, inspiration, and health, singing and preaching the glory of God to the many billions of intelligent body cells. At that stage of development one is really free, and is born free in succeeding incarnations if he wishes to return to dry the tears of others. Those who have attained this free-dom carry halos of invisible healing rays; wherever they go, they scatter the light of prosperity and health.

SUMMARY

In order to destroy ill health and failure we must dig be-neath the surface and get at their roots, which lie buried in the subconscious mind. Health and success or disease and

11

failure are the fruits of our actions not only in this life but in many lives. When the repeated efforts of an intelligent person to gain health or success miscarry, then disease and failure had their inception in past incarnations. Such chronic cases can be cured only by super-advanced methods of intuitional concentration and meditation.

True happiness and safety are realized by those who know how to destroy scientifically the hidden, ungerminated seeds of transgressions against the laws of physical, mental and spiritual health.

Super-Advanced Course No. 1

·•·✠·•·

Lesson No. 9

·•·✠·•·

UNIQUE CONCRETE PSYCHOLOGICAL MACHINES OR INNER DEVICES FOR CONQUERING FEAR, ANGER, GREED, TEMPTATION, FAILURE CONSCIOUS- NESS AND INFERIORITY COMPLEXES

By

SWAMI YOGANANDA

·•·✠·•·

This sacred lesson is meant only for the devoted Yogoda
student who would, untiringly and unceasingly,
seek God until he finds Him

·•·✠·•·

Published By
YOGODA SAT-SANGA SOCIETY
3880 San Rafael Avenue
Mount Washington
Los Angeles, Calif.

CONQUERING FEAR

Fear complexes.   When fear overpowers you, realize that nothing worse than physical death can happen to you; and if that does happen, it releases you from the object of your fears. Realize death is not a tyrant but a deliverer: it releases us from all physical pain and mental suffering. Death is the physical, mental and spiritual anodyne which brings relief from all anguish for a period immediately following mortal life.

Do not fear accidents and disease because you have recently encountered them. Such fear will create a disease and accident consciousness, and if it is strong enough you will draw to yourself the very things you most fear. On the other hand, fearlessness will in all probability avert them and minimize their power.

A mental indulgence in fear will create a subconscious fear habit. Thus, when something really upsetting to the regular routine occurs, the cultivated subconscious fear habit will assert itself, magnifying the object of our fears and paralyzing the will-to-fight-fear faculty of the conscious mind. Man is made in the image of God and has all the powers and potentialities of God; therefore, it is wrong for him to think that trials are greater than his divinity. Remember, no matter how great your trials may be, you are able to conquer them. God will not suffer you to be tempted and tried beyond your strength.

When fear comes, tense and relax—exhale several times. Switch on the currents of calmness and serenity. Let your whole mental machinery awaken and actively hum with the vibration of will to do something. Then harness the power

1

of will to the cogwheels of fearless caution and continuous good judgment, which in turn must constantly revolve and produce mental devices for escaping your specific impending calamity.

When something is threatening to injure you, do not throttle the all-producing inner machine of your consciousness by fear. Rather, use the fear as a stimulus to accelerate your inner machine of consciousness to produce some mental devices which will instantly remove the cause of fear. These mental devices to escape fear are so numerous that they have to be specially fashioned by the almighty tool of consciousness, according to the specific and extraordinary needs of an individual. When something is threatening you, do not sit idle—*do something about it calmly* mustering all the power of your will and judgment. Will is the motive power which works the machine of activity.

Fear should not produce mental inertia, paralysis, or despondency; instead, it should spur you on to calm, cautious activity, avoiding equally rashness and timidity.

Fear of failure or sickness is nourished by thinking constantly of all kinds of dire possibilities, until they take root in the subconscious and finally in the super-conscious. Then these fear seeds begin to germinate and fill the conscious mind with fear plants which bear poisonous, death-dealing, fear fruits.

Uproot fear from within by forceful concentration on courage—and by shifting your consciousness to the absolute peace within. After you succeed in uprooting fear psychologically, then focus your attention on methods for acquiring prosperity and health.

2

Associate with healthy and prosperous people who do not fear sickness or failure.

If you are unable to dislodge the haunting fear of ill health or failure, divert your mind by turning your attention to interesting, absorbing books, or even to harmless amusements. After the mind forgets its haunting fear, let it take up the shovels of different mental devices and dig out the causes and roots of failure and ill health from the soil of your daily life.

Fear aggravates all our miseries. It intensifies a hundred-fold our physical pain and mental agony.

Fear contaminates vivid imagination emotions, influencing the subconsciousness to such an extent that it in turn completely destroys the willing efforts of the consciousness.

Fear develops in an individual a malignant magnetism by which he attracts the very object of which he is afraid, as a magnet attracts a piece of iron or steel.

Fear is poison to both body and mind, *unless it is controlled and used as a stimulus* to calm caution.

Uncontrolled fear destroys business initiative. It paralyzes the desire to repeat success-producing efforts. Fear inhibits the almighty power of the soul. Have fear of nothing but fear itself.

Fear has a very deleterious effect on the heart, nervous system, and brain. It is destructive to mental initiative, courage, judgment, common sense, and to the will.

Fear throws a veil over intuition and robs you of your confidence to master your difficulties.

Kill fear by refusing to be afraid of it.

3

Know that you are safe behind the battlements of God's eternal safety, even though death knocks at your door or you are rocked on the seas of suffering. His protecting rays can dispel the menacing clouds of doomsday, calm the waves of trials and keep you safe, whether you are in a castle or on the open battlefield of life where bullets of trials are incessantly flying. Remember, without God's protection your life, health, and prosperity are in dire peril, even though you are locked in a scientifically hygienic castle of opulence, surrounded by impregnable moats, manned by all the fire-emitting guns of man.

CONQUERING ANGER

Anger makes you surly and contaminates others with the same sullenness. Anger makes *you* uncomfortable first and then it transmits your discomforts to others. Anger defeats its own purpose; it is not an antidote for anger. Violent wrath may bring suppression of a weaker wrath, but it will never *destroy* it.

Be calm and indifferent to those who deliberately enjoy making you angry.

Show outward anger only to those whom you can momentarily stupefy and thus prevent from doing mischief, but never initiate anger if it actually makes you angry—or, rather, never be angry *inwardly*. Anger poisons your own peace and that of others. Anger poisons calmness and blights understanding; in fact, it is the manna of misunderstanding. Anger is the method by which fools attempt to conquer others. Your anger merely rouses your enemy's wrath, and

4

you make him stronger and more powerful, instead of conquering him.

The antidote   Love is the great antidote for anger.
for anger.   Do not be demonstrative in your love for an angry person. He is not in the mood to appreciate it, his reasoning faculty and good nature being temporarily paralyzed. All you can do is to give him your good will. The expression of righteous indignation for the purpose of averting evil is, of course, productive of good.

Anger gives birth to jealousy, hatred, spite, vengefulness, destructiveness, "brain storms," temporary insanity leading to horrible crimes, and so forth.

When anger attacks you, *conquer it.* When you are angry, say nothing. Knowing it to be a disease (like a cold, for instance), throw it off by a mental warm bath. Fill your mind, to the exclusion of all else, with thoughts of those with whom you can never be angry, no matter what they do.

When violently angry, douse your head with cold water, or rub the medulla, the temples, the forehead (especially between the eyebrows), and the top of the head with a piece of ice.

Develop metaphysical reason in order to destroy anger. Look upon the anger-rousing agent as a child of God, a little five-year-old baby brother who has unwittingly, perhaps, stabbed you. You cannot wish to stab back this little brother who did not know what he was doing when he injured you. When you become Christ-like and look upon all humanity as little brothers hurting one another—"for they know not

5

what they do"—then you cannot feel angry with anyone. Ignorance is the mother of all anger.

Mentally destroy anger; do not permit it to poison your peace and disturb your habitual joy-giving serenity.

When anger comes, think of love; think that, as you do not want others to be angry with you, you do not wish others to feel your ugly anger.

When anger comes, set in motion your machinery of calmness; let it move the cogwheel of peace, love and forgiveness. And with these antidotes, *destroy anger*.

OVERCOMING GREED

Remember, you eat to live but do not live to eat. Greed is a servant of the palate—and enemy of digestion and health. Greed wants to please itself and the sense of taste at the cost of your happiness.

Greed produces evil habits of eating, utterly disregarding the needs of the body even to the point of death. Greed says: "Let us eat, drink, and be merry, for tomorrow we die!" Self-control in eating, good mastication, plain food and eating only when you are very hungry, develop right habits of eating and destroy greed. Self-control may not seem so alluring as self-indulgence, but it protects your health.

The purpose of self-restraint in eating is primarily the conservation of health, though wholesome food need not be, and certainly should not be, unpalatable. Eat often, eat less, think of your health and digestion, and do not concentrate on your palate, if you want to conquer greed.

6

Remember, greed for too many possessions is also evil. Greed for an increasingly greater number of material objects causes a person to disregard health, happiness and honest methods of earning a living. A greedy individual shatters his health and destroys his peace of mind by his self-indulgence. Such a person is never satisfied.

Concentrating on your *needs* is an antidote for your insatiable greed for money or possessions.

The noble ambition to acquire wealth in order to aid worthy causes is not greed—for it is not insatiable—it is always satisfied when it can help others.

OVERCOMING FAILURE

Uproot the consciousness of business failure. Three out of four business men in America fail: first, because they choose a wrong vocation; next, because they "give up" too quickly; and last, because their products lack quality.

An inferiority complex is born of contact with weak-minded people and the weak innate subconscious mind. A superiority complex results from false pride and an inflated ego. Both inferiority and superiority complexes are destructive to self-development. Both are fostered by imagination, ignoring facts, while neither belongs to the true, all-powerful nature of the soul. Develop self-confidence by conquering your weaknesses. Found your self-confidence on actual achievements, and you will be free from all inferiority and superiority complexes.

7

Super-Advanced Course No. 1

—+—

Lesson No. 10

THE ART OF SUPER-RELAXATION

—+—

By

SWAMI YOGANANDA

—+—

This sacred lesson is meant only for the devoted Yogoda
student who would, untiringly and unceasingly,
seek God until he finds Him

—+—

Published By
YOGODA SAT-SANGA SOCIETY
3880 San Rafael Avenue
Mount Washington
Los Angeles, Calif.

Super-relaxation is complete *voluntary* withdrawal of consciousness and energy from the entire body.

The soul has suffered itself to be lured away from the vast kingdom of the Spirit and to be trapped in the little, physical body. As the soul forsook its vast kingdom of Omnipresence, it passed through many smaller realms of life until it finally entered through the trapdoor of material attachment and found itself imprisoned in the body, unable to get out and return to its home of Omnipresence. The bird of paradise has become the bird encaged behind the prison bars of flesh. Hence, every soul prisoner who has walked through the gates of ideational, astral, and physical confinements into the trap of body consciousness must learn to open these inner prison gates before he can find freedom and return to the Spirit.

Physical culturists and other health enthusiasts, as well as spiritual teachers, often talk of relaxation; but few know how to achieve it.

Have you seen an electric bulb to which a dimmer device is attached? You can operate this device by moving a little rod backwards, thus gradually dimming the light in the bulb until it is almost extinguished. Then, if you return the rod to its first position, the light gradually becomes brighter until it resumes its original brilliancy. Hence, by means of the dimmer device, you can get several degrees of light in the bulb. For instance, starting with the dark bulb, moving the rod slightly each time results in (1) a very dim light, (2) a dim light, (3) a light of medium brightness, and (4) a bright light.

1

How to switch on, The body and mind also have dimmer
switch off, and devices. By using the first method, you
dim consciousness can relax your mind and switch off
and energy in energy from the body. This is known
the body. as *physical relaxation.* By using the
second method, you can shut out mental
distractions. This is called *mental relaxation.*

Some people know how to relax physically but not
mentally. To keep the mind fixed constantly on the soul
after freeing it from all distracting thoughts, is called *soul
relaxation.*

Mental relaxation signifies complete mental rest. You can
achieve this by practicing to go to sleep at will. Relax the
body and think of the drowsiness you usually feel just before
you fall asleep. Then try actually to reproduce that state.
(*Use imagination,* not will, to do this.) Most people do not
relax even while they sleep. Their minds are restless; hence
they dream. Therefore, conscious mental relaxation is better
than relaxation which is the by-product of physical passive
relaxation or sleep.[1] In this way you can either dream or
keep dreams off your mental moving-picture screen, as you
choose. No matter how busy you are, do not forget now
and then to free your mind completely from worries and all
duties. Just dismiss them from your mind. Remember, you
were not made for them; they were made by you. Do not
allow them to torture you. When you are beset by the
greatest mental trials or worries, try to fall asleep. If you
can do that, you will find, on awakening, that the mental

[1] Passive sensory relaxation, or sleep, comes automatically when the body
is tired. Conscious sensory relaxation is self-induced.

2

tension is relieved and that worry has loosened its grip on you. Just tell yourself that even if you die the earth would continue to follow its orbit, and business would be carried on as usual; hence, why worry? When you take yourself too seriously death comes along to mock you and remind you of the brevity of material life and its duties.

The mind must manifest calmness; where the worries and trials of everyday life are concerned, it must be like water which does not retain any impression of the waves that play on its bosom.

This is no brief for negligence in business, which should be avoided as carefully as the unnecessary concern arising from an inflated sense of responsibility. You are *not* too busy to eat, sleep, and relax. You must remember that material success, without health, peace and happiness, is of little value to you, for what does it avail you when you are seriously ill and die?

Therefore, "let go" of your worries. Enter into absolute silence every morning and night, and banish thoughts for several minutes each time. Then think of some happy incident in your life; dwell on it and visualize it; mentally go through some pleasant experience over and over again until you forget your worries entirely.

Mental relaxation consists in the ability to free the attention at will from haunting worries over past and present difficulties; consciousness of constant duty; dread of accidents and other haunting fears; greed; passion; evil or disturbing thoughts, and attachments. Mastery in mental relaxation comes with faithful practice. It can be attained by freeing the mind of all thoughts at will and keeping the attention fixed on the peace and contentment within.

By the third method you learn *super-relaxation*. Metaphysical super-relaxation consists in freeing the entire human consciousness from its identification with the body, money, possessions, name, fame, family, country, the world, and the human race and its habits. Super-relaxation consists in disengaging the attention by degrees from consciousness, subconsciousness, the semi-superconscious state of deep, restful sleep, the superconscious state felt after meditation, and Christ Consciousness[1], and identifying it completely with Cosmic Consciousness[2]. Mental relaxation and semi-super-relaxation consist in releasing consciousness from the delusion of duality and resting the mind, keeping it identified with one's own real nature of unity in Spirit. You have hypnotized yourselves into thinking you are human beings, whereas, in reality you are gods.

By the last and most important method, you learn scientifically to disengage your attention and energy from their identification with the world of sensations, muscles, heart,

[1] Signs of Christ Consciousness: Contacting others' thoughts and feelings instantaneously. Contacting places and their vibrations instantaneously. Contacting several planets and spheres instantaneously. If you want Christ Consciousness, do not look for phenomena, but march steadily on, deepening your meditation and your joy born of meditation. Do not be lured from your goal by psychical phenomena, no matter how marvelous they may seem. Love for everybody characterizes those who have Christ Consciousness. Through Christ Consciousness, others' feelings and different atmospheric and planetary conditions can be projected in your consciousness by merely thinking of them.

[2] Signs of Cosmic Consciousness: Beholding your consciousness as the only reality.

4

spine, etc. There are several kinds of this astral and mental relaxation.

Unconscious muscular relaxation. This is usually practiced in a very imperfect manner by moving the limbs. Those who use this method generally keep half of the muscles tensed and possibly the other half relaxed. Some remain completely tensed and only imagine they are relaxed.

Conscious muscular or motor relaxation. It is the purpose of this method of relaxation to withdraw consciousness and energy completely from the muscles. To achieve this, first gently tense the entire body or a certain body part. Then relax or withdraw all energy from the body or the body part in question and remain relaxed, *without the slightest physical motion.* The complete absence of motion and tension from muscles and limbs is true relaxation. Imagine that the body is jellylike, without bones or muscles. When you can do this, you have attained perfect muscular relaxation.

Passive sensory relaxation or sleep. In muscular relaxation, the mind and energy are relaxed or withdrawn from the muscles, but not from the sensory nerves or the sense-seats of optical, auditory, olfactory, tactual, and gustatory nerves. During deep sleep the mind and energy are passively and unconsciously withdrawn from the motor and sensory nerves, and even thoughts are banished. When the soul becomes satiated

5

with material contacts during the day, it passively switches off the life force and mind from the senses. Sleep can be induced at will, by suddenly relaxing the body, lying down on the back, dismissing all thoughts, and by closing the eyes. Try this until you learn to sleep or dream at will. With closed eyes, visualize a different room from the one in which you are resting and fall asleep thinking of it. In this manner dreams can be induced.

That which can be done passively and unconsciously can also be attained consciously. By practicing the fourth Yogoda lesson one can achieve complete calmness in the heart, lungs, and other inner organs. When the muscles and inner organs are freed from motion by relaxation, the breaking down of bodily tissues and decay are temporarily inhibited. This in turn helps to keep the blood stream pure, for when there is decay going on in the body, the waste products are thrown into, and poison, the venous blood.

When tissues stop decaying, the venous blood ceases to accumulate in the body. This gives the heart a much needed rest, for there is no longer any need of its pumping great quantities of venous blood into the lungs for purification, as the neutralized electrified tissues do not require blood and oxygen. Thus, heart action and breathing become unnecessary. This leads to the release of the enormous quantity of life current which otherwise would have been needed in the heart for the daily task of pumping eighteen tons of blood through the system. Thus, the many billions of cells no longer *work and move* through inner currents and are no

6

longer dependent on blood and oxygen. They *rest* and depend more and more on this inner sustaining current to enable them to live in a *conscious, suspended, undecaying state.* When the body cells learn the art of living without bread (blood and oxygen), they truly know how to live by the Word of God or the inner energy coming down from the medulla, and on the released currents from the heart and other inner organs.

When this energy is withdrawn from all inner organs, it is switched off scientifically and automatically from the sensory and motor nerves. This simultaneously insures (1) conscious sensory relaxation[1], and (2) conscious involuntary relaxation. When the energy is withdrawn from all the sensory nerves, the five sense-telephones are disconnected. No sensations can reach the brain and intelligence operators. The attention being thus shut off from sensations, it gains freedom from thoughts which have their inception in sensations, as well as the associated thoughts of the subconscious memory. This leaves the scientifically freed attention unhampered to march Godward. Sensory involuntary relaxation is meagerly possible by the unscientific method of mental diversion. Trying to free the attention by diverting it from sensations has been tried the world over with little or no success.

[1] Conscious sensory relaxation can be attained also by breathing in and out, followed by long, comfortable exhalations. Concentrate on breathlessness. Expel the breath every time you feel the desire to breathe, and rest attention on the breathless, comfortable state. By continuous inhalation and exhalation the blood becomes oxygenized, thus making breathlessness possible.

What is "death"?   Finally, *death* is not annihilation. It is the switching off of the nerve current from the entire body-bulb. *Death* is a state of passive involuntary relaxation brought on by sudden accidents, disease, or sorrow. The forcible, sudden, and permanent disconnection of life current from the body-bulb is popularly called *death* or complete annihilation of life. In reality it is only a temporary state—it is not the end of things, but merely the transfer from the domain of changeable, ugly matter to the realm of infinite joy and multicolored, flashing lights.

Why not learn the method by which you can switch off the life current from the entire body through conscious will by the steady, conscientious practice of the fourth Yogoda lesson, thus freeing the soul from the bondage of death. Besides, just as electricity does not die with the breaking of the bulb into which it flows but merely retires into the big dynamo behind it, so our real self is not destroyed but retires into the Infinite Omnipresent Self, when our life forces are switched off from the body-bulb. After thoroughly mastering the fourth lesson and attaining the breathless state, the following method will be found very helpful for inducing relaxation at will.

Method for inducing relaxation.   First, close eyes; expel breath; switch off attention and energy from the senses. Feel and mentally watch the heart and circulation and calm it down by the command of will as you stop a watch by gently touching its spring. With calmness you can arrest the activities of the entire physical machinery. Then switch on the current in the spine and

8

brain, disconnecting your current from the five sense-telephones. Convert your brain into a divine radio, catching the Cosmic Sound and the Song of God. Or you may switch off entirely the body and brain bulbs and merge with the Omnipresent Cosmic Dynamo. You can return at will, snatching yourself from the Infinite Omnipresence and switching on life in your body-bulb, thus caging your omnipresence there. Keep switching on and switching off the life current in the body until you know you are a part of the One Light which lights all the heavenly lamps of atoms, stars and all living creatures.

Those who know how to leave the body consciously can return to it consciously. People who die by accidents or are otherwise forced out of the body cannot re-enter it at will, but bodies under suspended animation can be reawakened by physical and mental methods.

Do not leave the body *by imagination;* learn to do it actually by releasing consciousness (1) from the muscles, and (2) from the senses by withdrawing the life force from the five sense-telephones. After sensory relaxation is achieved the heart calms down, and the consciousness and energy lodge themselves in the spine.

Involuntary relaxation consists in the ability to calm the heart at will and raise consciousness upward through the seven centers and out of the medulla into Infinite Spirit.

PRAYER AND SUMMARY

O Spirit, release my life and consciousness from possessions, from attachments. Release, Thou, my life and mind

9

from the tensed body, dimming consciousness and life-force from the body muscles. Release my consciousness from the senses, then from the breath; then unlock the energy and unconsciousness from the heart.

Then, O Spirit, lodge life and consciousness in the spine. And then release them unto the Spirit into Infinite Spaces. Oh, make me behold Milky Way Spiral Nebulae floating and glimmering in me.

Then, O Spirit, bring the bright Bird of Omnipresence back through its cage door of medulla into the passage of the spine; and then let it fly into the heart and sing vitality there. And then let it flutter its wings of breaths into the two lungs. And then, O Spirit, let it flutter at last over the walls of flesh.

Om . . . vibrate in the hands, in the feet, in the body, in the muscles! Om . . . vibrate in the spirit! Om . . . come back to the spine, back to the heart, and back to the muscles again!

Super-Advanced Course No. 1

◦◦⁂◦◦

Lesson No. 11

CONVERTING THE HANDS INTO HEALING BATTERIES OF LIFE FORCE:
HEALING LIKE JESUS BY THE LAYING ON OF HANDS
HEALING STRICKEN PEOPLE FROM A DISTANCE

By

SWAMI YOGANANDA

◦◦⁂◦◦

This sacred lesson is meant only for the devoted Yogoda
student who would, untiringly and unceasingly,
seek God until he finds Him

◦◦⁂◦◦

Published By
YOGODA SAT-SANGA SOCIETY
3880 San Rafael Avenue
Mount Washington
Los Angeles, Calif.

The body's sources The human body may be compared to
of energy. the wet battery of an automobile. Just
as the proper functioning of an automo-
bile battery depends upon distilled water from without and
energy from within, so the proper functioning of the human
body battery depends upon food from without and life force
from within.

Will draws energy This life force is stored mainly in the
from the cosmos medulla and distributed through the sub-
into the body. dynamos in the five plexuses. The
medulla is fed by conscious Cosmic
Energy which surrounds the body and which is drawn into
the body by the power of the will.

Cosmic Energy is converted into life force by the will
which is the radio as well as the main dynamo of the body.
Very often, however, people become discouraged and permit hereditary inhibitions in the subconscious mind to
hamper the will. The suggestions of old age, accidents,
diseases, heredity, instincts, etc., demoralize the will in many
individuals. During a serious illness, for instance, memories
of previous ailments as well as memories of past failures,
frustrations, and disappointments which were due to weakness, fill consciousness with the fear that the body cannot recover. Death occurs if one "gives up"; if he refuses to be
disheartened, the will produces life force which can repair
and remodel all tissues, including bones, organs, etc. Therefore, if one refuses to become discouraged or to take seriously illusive body changes and thoughts of hereditary

limitations, bodily disintegration is arrested. Different degrees of will power develop corresponding degrees of sensitiveness to pain or death. Some combat injuries and live; others resign themselves "to their fate" at the slightest indisposition. Thus it becomes evident that the duration of life is dependent upon the will.

Many people die mentally long before they die physically. When one ceases to have ambitions and to be interested in life, the will becomes paralyzed. When this will-radio is untuned or destroyed, Cosmic Energy ceases to supply the reserve dynamo of the medulla, and physical health slowly fails from want of life force. This is the principal cause for the symptoms of old age. *The stronger the will, the greater the flow of energy into the tissues and body parts.*

Will is the life-sustaining factor. Food cannot rejuvenate the body of an individual whose will is weak, for it is the inner energy, or life force, which converts food into energy. Solids, liquids, and gases cannot be assimilated after the supply of life force, which is dependent upon the will, has ceased. When one has a strong, unflinching will, he grows more and more independent of food. He can absorb the consciousness of changelessness and inject it with Cosmic Energy into all the cells, making them neutral and free from decay or growth. Then these cells become electrified and live only by the vibratory power of intelligent Cosmic Energy, or the Word of God (which is God according to the Bible).

Thoughts of Cosmic Energy, through the will, *fatigue shut off the* feeds the medulla which in turn feeds *supply of energy.* the five plexuses. The life force in the plexuses carries on the telephonic work of the five senses through the sensory nerves and of the muscles and joints through the motor nerves. The same life principle charges the circulation, vitalizes each blood cell, and also feeds every nerve, all of which in turn recharge the other cells of the body. As the cells are but condensed will and energy, they can be instantaneously renewed by the power of strong, unflinching will. Therefore, one should never say or think he is tired, for by doing that one becomes twice as tired and paralyzes the will which must be active in order to draw Cosmic Energy into the body.

Acute and chronic diseases result from lack of life force, a faulty diet, overwork, or other bad habits.

Medicine cannot Food and medicine have but an indi- *affect the mental* rect, limited effect on the simple germ *behavior and* cells, and are very slow to change the *"disease notions"* nature and behavior of the somatic cells *of the somatic cells.* and specialized organs. Medicine and the proper food can bring about many cures, but they cannot recreate an organ. Why? The sperm and ovum, drawing nutrition from the mother's body, develop from boneless specks of protoplasm into a baby with hard bones and nerves and organs, etc. Life force and food created all the specialized organs from the sperm and

3

ovum, because they contained the mind-obeying germ cells. However, as the organs were formed, the cells changed. It is because these changed (somatic) cells, constituting the organs, are very unyielding and hard to control that food and chemicals are unable to recreate organs. Originally, mind and life force induce the germ cells to create organs, but once the germ cells change into somatic cells they begin to rule the mind and life force. Hence humanity can regain the power to recreate lost limbs, organs, etc., only by learning to convert the somatic cells back to their original obedient germ-cell state. By freeing life force and mind from bodily slavery, by increasing vitality and mental power, the somatic cells can be made to change into germ cells.

Why do germ cells change into obstinate somatic cells? The vital organs are maintained and guided by the subconscious mind which contains the record of our experiences and behavior throughout all incarnations. Therefore, though the human body develops from changeable germ cells, subconscious, fixed designers slowly transform these germ cells into somatic cells which make up the specialized organs and limbs of the human body. In other words, the somatic cells are governed by specialized organic designers. These are the result of our past actions, and are born and die with the organs and limbs which they consciously design and build. When one of the lungs or an arm is lost, the specialized designer in that lung or arm dies with it. Therefore, the body is unable to recreate these lost body parts.

4

Can lost organs,   In order to recreate lost organs, etc.,
limbs, etc., be   the following is necessary:
recreated?   (1) The life force must be made to
                                 obey the will instantaneously;
(2) The will must be changed to all-creating Divine
    Will;
(3) The life force must be supplied with psychological
    designers of human organs when such organs are
    lost through disease or accident. One must visual-
    ize a lost designer until it is born again. To be
    able to do that, one must know how to materialize
    thoughts;
(4) The will must be able to float them in the life
    force, and the life force must be charged continu-
    ously with Cosmic Energy. The will must be
    kept free from, and unhampered by, discouraging
    hereditary suggestions;
(5) Lastly, when the will can overcome all hereditary
    instinctive prejudices regarding the recreation of
    human organs, and create living psychological
    designers, then these designers begin to use the
    extra charge of life energy and condense the semi-
    conscious life force into electrons which are further
    condensed into gases, etc. Then the designers
    begin to use the new protoplasm created by con-
    densation of energy, food chemicals, and blood
    from the body, to recreate and replace a lost organ.
Buried in the human mind is the evil, weak suggestion of
powerlessness of millions of years, and it will take years to
learn how to put the above methods into practice.

The efficacy of medical healing methods is limited, as other methods are. Therefore, scientific healing can be effected unfailingly by the development and strengthening of will power and life force. Moreover, this human will power must be impregnated with the invincible, all-creating, unlimited healing power of the Almighty. Neither medicine nor any other material agency has managed to obtain control over the electronic, vibratory force and recreating power of the body cells. If the body is deprived of energy and consciousness, it cannot live. There is no denying that *materia medica* has its uses. However, the more you depend on the limited power of drugs, the weaker your will and access to God's unlimited healing power, and the more you depend on God, the less *need* you depend on drugs. Organic defects and chronic diseases can be dealt with successfully through divinely charged will power and life force, which alone are the almighty creators and rebuilders of all new or decayed body tissues. Bones, blood, marrow, nerves, brain tissues— everything in the body is directly materialized out of the sperm by the latent will power and life force.

Adam and Eve reproduced themselves by materializing will and energy. Of course, originally Divine Will had to create especially, and materialize, human sperm and ovum, and these contained God's most perfect design. The primeval sperm cells and ova were materialized into the organism of the original man and woman, Adam and Eve, before propagation

6

by the law of cause and effect was instituted. They could re-create their bodies, and propagate themselves, by materializ-ing their vitality and tendencies and clothing them with materialized limbs and flesh. They were in constant com-munion with the Almighty. Therefore, their will force was in tune with the Infinite Will, and they could create human beings out of the ether in the same manner as God. Only after their will became subservient to the ego and the senses, instead of being guided by wisdom, did they develop sex and sex creation. This was their fall from heavenly powers to earthly ways of creation and living. Their will, no longer guided by wisdom, opposed the Divine Will which is guided by wisdom only. Ever since, misguided, obstinate self-will and satanic ignorance—being concentrated on the change-able body instead of the unchangeable, infinite Spirit in the body—have created defective, limited mental designers of bodies and their organs. These defective mental designers, inherited from the original erring parents of all humanity, are thus perpetuated in the countless human sperm cells and ova. In this manner did man lose the power to materialize spiritual children and to create perfect bodies in which any organ or limb, etc., could be recreated at will.

The breaking of bones, the loss of limbs or organs, or even injury or loss of the brain would be of no consequence if they could be restored or recreated painlessly by super-conscious methods and Divine Will, during conscious relaxa-tion or under anesthesia. The territory of the will and energy is the entire human body. The ordinary individual

7

who is a slave to his body finds that he has only imperfect control over the muscles.

First learn to control the muscles and the body by will and life force; then learn to feel the living relation between will and life force and the vital organs by relaxation of the sensory nerves and involuntary organs, *i.e.*, by "switching off" energy from heart, lungs, etc. *The purpose of tension and relaxation is dissociation of life force and mind from the consciousness of the body.* When that is accomplished, the will and life force actually own the whole body and can, through their healing rays, remove chronic defects from any body part.

The astral body, in appearance like a vast nebula or the tail of a comet, charges the physical body with Cosmic Energy through the medulla.

As material science has demonstrated that a piece of chicken heart can be kept alive and growing by the administration of food and chemicals, so Hindu Yoga has shown that the human body and heart can be kept alive in a suspended state, without food, oxygen, or chemicals.[1]

By practicing the exercises given in the second Yogoda lesson, one can learn, with absolute faith in the almighty power of will, slowly, conscientiously, and patiently to tense and relax, *i.e.*, alternately to put forth and withdraw life force, several times, from any body part that is diseased.

[1]If the heart were stopped and energy distributed throughout the body, the latter would not decompose; but if the heart were stopped and energy withdrawn from the spine, bodily decay would be inevitable. Yogis know how to stop heart and lung action voluntarily yet keep physically alive by retaining some Cosmic Energy in their bodies to sustain the cells in a suspended state.

A body part may be recharged without tension. This method is not effective for the involuntary organs which can be recharged only by practicing the fourth Yogoda lesson. In order to heal cardiac or cerebral disorders, one may send energy mentally to the affected area by merely concentrating on it, without tensing. By this method one can send a feeble current of energy to any body part. Actually tensing with will, of course, produces more energy than concentration alone, but very gentle conscious tension and relaxation of the whole body also sends healing energy, vitality, etc., to heart and brain. It must be remembered, however, that in tensing and relaxing the whole body with a view to curing heart or brain disorders concentration must be centered on the affected organ.

There is also another method of healing:

Sit erect. Gently tense and relax the whole body. Calm yourself. Touch the medulla once, in order to make it easier for you to concentrate on it. Then visualize Cosmic Energy surrounding and entering the body through the medulla and at the point between the eyebrows, and pouring into the spine. Feel the energy flowing down the whole length of the two arms into the hands. Continue tensing and relaxing and feeling the life force flow from the medulla and the point between the eyebrows through the spine to the hands. Then stop tensing and relaxing, and firmly rub the entire bare left arm with the right palm (up and down, several times). Do the same to the right arm with the left palm. Then relax, continuously visualizing and willing Cosmic Energy to descend from the medulla through

9

the arms into your hands. Now, with closed eyes, rapidly but gently rub your palms together about twenty times. Then separate the hands, and lift the arms upward. You will feel the life current flowing from the medulla into the spine, especially through both arms and hands, with a pricking, tingling sensation.

Your energy-magnetized hands may be used either for curing any diseased part of your own body or some other person's who need not be in your immediate vicinity, for it is not necessary to touch your patient. This life force passing through your hands has infinite power of projection.

The human will and energy imperfectly control the human body, but the divinely transmitted will can work perfectly, not only in healing your own physical ailments, but also those of others, even though they be far away. You must, however, visualize your patient, and he must have faith in you. You must broadcast the healing force by moving your hands, electrified by the above method, up and down in space while willing the current to pass over your patient's diseased body part. Do this in a quiet room for fifteen minutes until you feel that you have accomplished your object.

Convert yourself into a divine battery, sending out through your hands divine healing rays whenever and wherever they may be needed. Then your hands, charged with divine power, will throw healing rays into your patient's heart and brain. Thus his seeds of ignorance will be destroyed, and he will smile with the health of God-love.

SUMMARY

Learn to convert your hands into healing batteries, so that divine currents will flow through them at will. Through this means when properly administered diseases of body and mind, as well as the malady of soul ignorance, have vanished under this benign touch, whether administered at close quarters or from afar. Thus one becomes the fisherman of souls, that he may catch them in the net of his divine healing wisdom and present them unto God.

Super-Advanced Course No. 1

Lesson No. 12

ESTHETIC WAY OF DEVELOPING

COSMIC CONSCIOUSNESS

By

SWAMI YOGANANDA

Published By
YOGODA SAT-SANGA SOCIETY
3880 San Rafael Avenue
Mount Washington
Los Angeles, Calif.

ESTHETIC WAY OF DEVELOPING
COSMIC CONSCIOUSNESS

Extending the   In feeling God, you must extend the
kingdom of heart territory of your feelings. You feel for
from your own your own heart; now you must every
to others.   day begin to feel more and more at one
         with the hearts of others, their woes,
struggles, joys and weal. To feel others' hearts means not
only that you must remain absorbed in loving and working
for yourself, but you must learn to work and spend for
others, protect and love others with the same degree of
interest and enthusiasm as for yourself.

See God in those Begin to feel interest and helpfulness
who hate you. and love toward one soul today, another
         tomorrow, another day after tomorrow.
And let these feelings be active, not weakly passive. Try to
love and help others *actively* each day, especially those who
love you. Keep on doing this until you can do it even to
those who care nothing for you. And at last let the feeling
of love and good will and helpfulness go forth to enfold even
those who hate you. This is the real, practical way by which
the soul can spread its victories from heart to heart, ever en-
larging its boundaries, until at last it can recover its rightful
kingdom of all the hearts of all creatures.

1

Feeling all hearts, you will feel the One Heart of God. Your unceasing love and unselfish readiness to help others without distinction of sex, creed or caste will make your heart big enough to receive all humanity therein. And once the love of all human beings and all living things shall have entered into your heart, your heart will be the One Heart of God. Feeling all hearts as one, you will feel the One Cosmic Heart beating behind all hearts. Recognizing no individual selfish love, feeling the same love for all, you will feel the One Great Love which is everlasting and forever burns as pure white flame on the universal altar of all hearts. Say silently to your own soul: "I shall drink Thy Love alone from all cups, O God! From the gold and silver and crystal cups of the world and from the shining invisible cups of human hearts, I shall drink Thy Love alone!"

Help yourself in the forms of others. Recognizing the God-love burning in all heart lamps, you will see and feel only God-love flowing through everybody and everything. Every time you meet a receptive human being, demonstrate by actions; and then make him feel your interest in his physical, mental and spiritual welfare. *Never neglect to do whatever you can for yourself in the forms of others.* To know the Spirit, you must become the Spirit and find yourself as manifested through the bodies and minds of others. Make the bubble of ego one with the ocean of Spirit. Make it big, so big that you can behold all the bubbles of living beings floating in it. Break the

2

boundaries of the small selfishness and include in boundless unselfishness all living beings, universes—everything ever created in the past, existing in the present, and to be created in the future.

Chant the Song of Cosmic Consciousness:

"So be Thou, my Lord,
Thou and I, never apart;
Wave of the sea,
Dissolve in the sea!
I am the bubble;
Make me the Sea!"

(From Whispers From Eternity.)

Break the walls of selfishness and make your love broad and deep enough to hold all humanity. The transcendental, metaphysical technique of developing Cosmic Consciousness.

But the quicker and more effective way is to add to the above methods of self-expansion the transcendental way of contacting Spirit. Often, during the day or night, close your eyes and peer into the fathomless eternity, above, beneath, on the right, on the left, and all around you, and say: "I am glad I turned my gaze from beholding and identifying myself with the little bubble of my body to the ocean of Infinity, hiding just behind the dark screen of my human vision."

Chant in silence to your soul: "Om . . . Om . . . Om!" And sing over and over and over, the Song of Cosmic Consciousness:

"So be Thou, my Lord,
Thou and I, never apart;
Wave of the sea,
Dissolve in the sea!
I am the bubble;
Make me the Sea!"

Keep on mentally racing millions of miles in all directions
at the same time, like an Aurora Borealis, until all directions
about you become tangibly shining and glimmering with the
searchlight rays of Infinite Light and Bliss.

Feel that as the very essence of your being. That is Cosmic
Consciousness.

Get out of the little cage of optical illusion of the body
with its confining cage bars of sensation.

Little bird of paradise, forget the familiar cage to which
you are so attached; behold your vast kingdom of Light and
Bliss hidden behind the shade of darkness which temporarily
shrouds your spiritual mental eye during the time you have
closed your physical eyes.

The Light shines   Daily seeing the material sunlight, you
behind darkness.   are blinded and unable to see the magic
                    world of eternally spread luminous elec-
trons shining behind the darkness born of closed eyes. Open
your eyes, O blind one! See how tiny your bird of ego is.
Now close your physical eyes and keep your spiritual eyes
wide open in the sunlight of a new understanding. See how
big YOU are, spread over Infinity and Eternity.

4

The hidden Cos- Listening to little, incomplete vibrations,
mic Sound. you have forgotten to float in the ocean
of Cosmic Sound. The Cosmic Song is
hidden behind the multitudinous little noises of your own
voice and the voices of material noises. The "still, small
voice" is never silent, but it cannot be heard for the clamor
drowning it. And all about us, everlastingly, night and day,
is playing the transcendental Music of the Spheres. "Seeing,
ye see not; hearing, ye hear not."

Lift the veils of Stop beholding only the little toy-
light and thought show of this world; close your physical
and behold God. eyes and plunge behind the screen of
darkness. Lift the veil of silence, and be-
hold the magic of soothing, rolling fires of planets, of trillions
of multicolored dancing atoms. Behold life-force dancing in
the hall of electrons. Behold one layer of light lying within
another. Behold consciousness dancing in the sphere of living
light. Behold the Bliss-God and His blessed angels dancing in
the thought-fashioned, wisdom-lighted Eternal Chamber of
Perpetual, ever-new Bliss. Lift all curtains of light and behold God in the glory of bliss. The Spiritual Eye is the
tunnel through all veils of light, leading straight to God.

Good habits ver- Human habits of beholding yourself as
sus human habits. the little body and its small playhouse of
No matter how the world, must be displaced by God
long you have habits. Human habit keeps reminding
erred, there is you of the little, unreal happiness of
hope for you. name, fame, territory and tiny, laugh-

5

ably valueless possessions. *Possess the Universe,* for the whole Universe is yours, O Prince of all Possessions! Forsake the slums of the beggar-ego and its pitiful claims to its tinsel kingdom of material beggary, O Prince-Image of God! Never mind even if you must live for a few incarnations in the slum of matter, becoming attached to its mirage of reality. Never mind what length of time you have spent and must still spend identified with matter. All of the ages past are as nothing compared to the Eternity of Time before you, that you may spend in the Bosom of God in the full and conscious possession of all His Glory. No matter how long you have erred and side-tracked away from God, you may NOW forsake the no-longer-attractive slums of ego and reclaim your kingdom of Divine Bliss in Eternity.

Taste God honey-combed in every-thing. The little centuries of human years are but days, nay, but a few hours in God's consciousness. Awaken! Arise from dreams of littleness to the realization of the vastness within you. You are dreaming you are a big moth, buzzing around the poisoned honey of blossoming sense-lures. Come! I will show you, my beloved, that you are the Eternal Fire which is drinking with countless mouths the Nectar-Bliss hidden in the honeycombs of all hearts and all things. God is honeycombed in everything. Drink Him through all noble experiences.

Revive your Omnipresent habits. Feed no longer your human habits with delusive human actions. Let them slowly starve for want of the food of

6

activity. Now, come! Meditate daily, with earnestness and devotion. Love God without ceasing. Thus may your Omnipresent habit-nature be revived in your consciousness, displacing the body-bound, sense-limited, world-caged human ideas, beliefs, and conscious and subconscious habits of earth life of this and past incarnations.

Love God through   Drink the nectar of God-love in all
all hearts.   hearts. Poison the veins of body attach-
                     ments, all small world-attachments. *Use every heart as your own wine cup from which to drink the fresh ambrosia of God-love. Drink not this Divine Love from one heart only, but drink freely from all hearts the love of God alone.*

Feel God as joy   Learn to love God as the joy felt in
of meditation.   meditation. Victory is very near. Only
Think of Him in   choose good paths before you start the
every action.   race to the goal of realization. Then
                     think of God as you start on the path of your material or spiritual duty. Then think of God with each footfall of your advancing feet as you make your way carefully and joyously over the broadening road of fulfill-ment. Then think of Him after you have traveled far on your life's path and finished your progressive action. Ask God to be with you when you, by your own will, choose good action. Then think of God before you eat body-nourishing food; then think of Him while you are eating it. Then, when you have finished eating, think of God.

Keep centered in God, instead of in matter. When you act in the world, forgetting God, you have changed your center from God to matter. And this grafted material nature will throw you into the whirlpool of change and will stifle you with worries and sorrows. Now revert to your own *real* nature. Change your center from material desires to desire for God. These material nature beggaries are only your grafted nature, so the only way you can forget these is to remember God as Peace and Bliss in your heart always. Ask God to make your peace, silence, joy and meditation His holy altars, where your soul may meet and commune with Him in the Holy of Holies. Let your prayer be: "Make my understanding the temple of Thy guidance."

Be silently drunk with God, but lose not your balance. Invoke God as Power in the temple of consciousness during the day. Let every action and every word that you utter be tinged and tipsy with God-love intoxication. Talk and act sensibly as a man who drinks a lot and yet keeps his senses awake and in command. Be drunk with God and let every action of your daily life be a temple of God's memory. Perform every action to please Him; and in the indestructible shrine of your devotion God will glisten in every thought.

Carry your love of God deep in your heart before you sleep. Cradle it there, so that when you dream you may dream of Him as resting on the fragrant altar of sleep, as Krishna or Christ or Peace or Bliss. In the temple of Sleep or Dreams, feel God as Peace or as ever-new Bliss. Actually,

8

God embraces you on His Bosom as Peace and Joy when you go to sleep in your subconscious chamber or your temple of dreams. Then you are sleeping locked in His Arms of Tranquillity. So, before you fall asleep, realize that you are going to embrace Him in sleep and dreams.

And when you are deeply sleeping or meditating, feel Him embracing you as the Omnipresent Bliss. The Great Omnipresence touches you in sleep and in meditation, and through His Bliss-touch He wants to make you forget your little, painful, worrying memories, mental and physical aches and spiritual agonies, which you garnered during your truant stay in the slums of matter.

Enthrone peace and joy in your heart. Feel that joy, no matter whom you meet and no matter what you do. If you can do this, though the universe shatter itself into nothingness or your soul or body be torn by trials, you will find Him dancing in your memory forever and forever. Let pure Joy dance in your memory, and God will dance with you.

Hold fast to your once lost spiritual treasure of joy. Now that it is regained, increase it by giving it freely to others and generously investing it in other hearts. Remember that whatsoever we selfishly keep for self is lost; and whatsoever we freely give in love to others, that treasure cannot be lost but yields its ever-increasing harvest of happiness, world without end. Worry and selfishness are highwaymen on the roadways of life, and they hold us up and rob us of our wealth of joy and peace. So, determine to hold fast to joy, no matter if death shall frown at your doors or your own subconscious mind may tell you that "all is lost." Drown all confusing noises in the silent, sweet harmony of your perfect, invincible joy.

Enthrone joy in the sanctuary of all your aspirations, your noble ambitions, noble actions, noble thoughts. And then you will feel God consciously as Joy reigning in the Kingdom of your Soul, governing every thought, every feeling and every memory, and laying His scepter on the white altar of your dreams to make every thought and every feeling and every memory a flower blooming there.

Remember this, my beloved: With her veil of sleep and peace, Mother Divine wipes away the dark sorrows of her ignorance-besmirched children. Go then to your dreams as a child to its mother's arms. Divine Love will be enshrined in all your memories of past incarnations and present thoughts. And then you will find that evil and misery were only your own imaginary dream-creations. You slept and dreamed a nightmare of evil; you awake in God and feel only joy and good existing everywhere.

And when the divine memory of constant joy shall arise on the Resurrection Day of your soul's return to its inheritance, you will forget forever your self-created nightmares of evil, and will behold with clear eyes the perfect beauty and good-ness that exists everywhere, because God is everywhere.

And then you will pray the only prayer that I pray for myself: "Heavenly Father, may Thy love shine forever on the shrine of my devotion. May my devotion for Thee for-ever burn on the altar of my memory, and may I be able to kindle love for Thee on all altar-hearts."

10

God-reminding action. New conception of Cosmic Consciousness in daily life.

1. Think of God before choosing an action. Think of Him before performing an action. And think of Him after the action is performed.

2. Feel God as love in all hearts. Feel God in the impartial love you feel for all human beings and in the tender love you feel for all created things.

3. Create God-like habits by thinking of Him as beauty and fragrance in the flowers; color in the rainbow; love, wisdom and power in all human minds; and vastness in the ocean and skies. Think of Him as life in the breeze; vitality in the sunshine; as peace in the moonbeams; reason in the mind; rest in dreams; joy in sleep; perennial, ever-new Bliss in meditation, and as love in all hearts. This is when the real comfort is found.

4. Reason God as energy which has frozen itself into electrons, gases, liquids and solids. Reason, think and act God as frozen Intelligent Energy.

5. Hear in all songs the heart-stirring ecstasy of God's song. Tune in—hear God's radio program of celestial inspirations.

6. Feel God in the temple of each thought that is born within your mind, in every feeling born within your heart, every aspiration born within your soul.

7. Enthrone God in the temple of Bliss in Meditation.

8. Feel the tangible God as that ever-burning Flame of joy which you directly feel within yourself.

Every step of the way, God walks by your side, speaking

to you in every breeze that blows, in every rippling river that goes singing to the sea.

O Divine Mother! Why need we ever cry: "Where art Thou?" Thou art eloquent everywhere, and Thy seeking children may glimpse Thee through windows of beauty, if they but lift to seeing eyes a single fragrant petal of a rose!

> Door of my heart
> Open I keep for Thee.
> Wilt Thou come, wilt Thou come?
> If but for once, come to me!
> Come to me, oh, come to me!

ALWAYS SING

> I will sing Thy name,
> I will drink Thy name,
> And get all drunk,
> Oh, with Thy name!

> I will sip Thy name,
> I will drink Thy name.
> Oh, thirstily and greedily
> I will drink Thy name.

> I will drink Thy name,
> I will give Thy name.
> I will spread Thy name,
> Oh, everywhere.

We will sing Thy name,
We will drink Thy name.
We'll dance and we'll sing
As we drink Thy name.

We'll sing Thy name
And drink Thy name,
And get all drunk,
Oh, with Thy name.

We'll dance through hearts,
We'll dance through lives,
And sing Thy name,
And sing Thy name.